Nursing: An Exquisite Obsession

Acknowledgements

The photos of Rhodri Morgan (p. 10) and of Swansea University (p. 101) are reproduced courtesy of Swansea University. The photo of Guys Hospital (p. 65) is reproduced courtesy of Guy's and St Thomas' NHS Foundation Trust. The photos of RCN Head Office (p. 129) and the RCN coat of arms (p. 167) are reproduced by kind permission of RCNi. The figure on p. 164 is reproduced by kind permission of the Royal College of Nursing. The photo of Gretta Styles (p. 208) is reproduced courtesy of the International Council of Nurses.

The publishers and author would like to thank Emap Publishing Ltd for kind permission to reproduce extracts from the *Nursing Times* on p. 51 and p. 88; Bauer Media Group for kind permission to reproduce the section from *Mother and Baby* on p. 53; Middlesex University for kind permission to reproduce the quote on p. 83; Manchester University Press for kind permission to reproduce the quote on p. 119; the Royal College of Nursing for permission to reproduce text from the RCN response to the consultation on primary health care initiated by the UK health departments (p. 149) and the Letter from the Chair of the IN Forum (p. 190); and BMJ Publishing Group for kind permission to reproduce the quote on p. 151.

Nursing:
an Exquisite Obsession

by

Professor Dame June Clark
DBE PhD RN FRCN FAAN FLSW

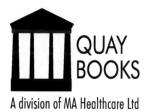

QUAY
BOOKS

A division of MA Healthcare Ltd

Quay Books Division, MA Healthcare Ltd,
St Jude's Church, Dulwich Road, London SE24 0PB

British Library Cataloguing-in-Publication Data
A catalogue record is available for this book

© MA Healthcare Limited 2016

ISBN-13: 978 1 85642 509 4

Printed by Mimeo, Huntingdon, Cambridgeshire

Contents

DEDICATION

For my husband Roger who has been at my side through thick and thin for more than fifty years.

And for my children, Andrew and Gillian, who I hope may be as proud of me as I am of them.

ACKNOWLEDGEMENTS

Very little in my nursing career, including this book, has been planned. But I have been fortunate to have had wonderful mentors throughout my nursing career and in preparing this book. It was Margretta Styles, one of my best loved mentors, who first said 'Nursing is for me an exquisite, excruciating obsession' and thus supplied the title of this book and its final chapter: as it was for her, so it has been for me. It was Norma Lang who helped me to understand that 'If you can't name it, you can't control it, finance it, teach it, research it, or put it into public policy' and challenged me to think about and articulate my understanding of 'this thing called nursing'. These two people have provided inspiration and the intellectual challenge that has driven my thinking about nursing ever since I first met them at the International Council of Nurses in 1990.

Other mentors also have greatly influenced my life in nursing, and therefore this book; they are no longer with us but their memory lives on in me and in the many others who benefited from their wisdom. In particular I owe a huge debt to Baroness Jean McFarlane, Marjorie Simpson, Grace Owen, Trevor Clay, Bob Tiffany, Monica Baly and Dame Sheila Quinn. What all these had in common was that like me, they 'burned for nursing' and were willing to share with me their vision of how nursing could and should be.

Without the encouragement and editorial skills of Rebecca Linssen and Charlotte Lindsay of Quay Books the manuscript would never have become a book: the first task, delegated to Charlotte, was to cut what I had written by 50%! A major source has been journal articles that I wrote, some nearly half a century ago; in some cases I still have the originals, but for others the RCN librarians did some wonderful detective work in the RCN library archives.

Dame Betty Kershaw and David Rye who lived with me through the good years and some of the bad years in the RCN read some of the earlier drafts, and moderated some of my more extreme comments.

But the biggest debt is to the hundreds, maybe thousands, of nurses both in the UK and around the world, whose lives have touched mine, and from whom I have learnt so much.

PREFACE

Several years ago Dame Sheila Quinn, who had just published her own autobiography, suggested that I should write mine. At the time I dismissed the idea as mere self-indulgence, and in any case I was far too busy. But one of the pleasures of growing older, and having time for such things, is coming across old photos, ancient yellowing press cuttings and other memorabilia, and remembering old times. The storeroom under our stairs is stuffed with boxes of papers and photos, which I should have thrown out but somehow couldn't bear to. Christmas cards from old friends often carried the message 'Do you remember when...', and as I found myself moving from my dotage into 'anecdotage', sharing memories about past escapades more and more provoked the response 'You ought to write a book about it!'

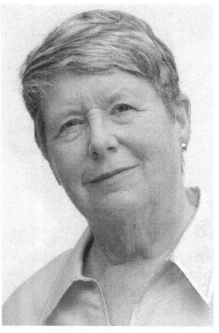

I was also increasingly concerned that today's nursing issues were exactly the same as those that had happened in the past, but that the profession seemed to have lost its corporate memory of them. When *A Voice for Nurses: A history of the Royal College of Nursing* was published in 2007 I was disappointed to find that it stopped at 1990. It seemed that the period since that time was very poorly documented and unlikely to be adequate for any future historian. In view of the radical change that was taking place in the Royal College of Nursing at that time I felt it was important that it should be documented and, in the words of the Welsh comedian Max Boyce, 'I was there'. For my own experience of events at that time, I found, as I have found many times before, that writing about it was cathartic and comforting. It was 'for my eyes only'; there was at that time no thought of publication.

Some time later I was asked to review the autobiography of another old friend, Mary Spinks. At her suggestion I sent what I had written to her publisher, asking, rather tentatively, whether it might be suitable for publication. Quay Books publisher, Rebecca Linssen, encouraged me to complete the manuscript and submit it. So I did.

I hope that readers will enjoy my story and perhaps relate it to their own experiences. But I hope also that my account of the development of the Royal College of Nursing during the last years of the 20th century and the early years of the 21st will be useful for understanding how and why the Royal College of Nursing has changed over the past decade and will therefore be a small contribution to its next history.

'Nursing is for me an exquisite, excruciating obsession'
Margretta Styles
On nursing: Toward a new endowment

PROLOGUE

'Nursing is for me an exquisite, excruciating obsession'
Styles MM (1982) *On Nursing: Toward a New Endowment.*

It is often said that in Wales everyone knows everybody else and that half of the population is related to the other half. It is a cultural characteristic that in any new meeting, for example in the taxi from the station to home, the first exchange will not, as in England, be 'What is your job?', but 'Where do you come from?' Very soon the participants will have shared the most intimate details of their life histories and their family trees.

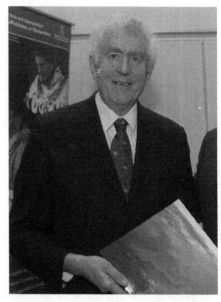

Rhodri Morgan, formerly First Minister of Wales, Chancellor Swansea University

It happened at a nursing conference dinner in 2001, which was hosted by the (then) new Chief Nursing Officer for Wales, Rosemary Kennedy. The guest of honour was Rhodri Morgan, the (then) newly-elected First Minister of Wales, and I was seated next to him. Never one to miss such an opportunity, I bent his ear about a number of issues, but in particular about the decision that we had recently made that in future all student nurses in Wales would be educated to degree level. The decision was fiercely resisted in many quarters (the precursor of the 'too posh to wash, too clever to care' debates which continue more than a decade later), and I wanted him to understand what we were doing and why.

Whenever I argue the case for undergraduate education for nurses, I refer to the row I had with my father when I was 18 years old and about to leave school. I had been offered a place to read Classics at University College London, subject to achieving the right grades in my A level exams, but I did not think I had done very well and was not going to try again but was going to Cardiff Royal Infirmary to be a nurse.

In the Welsh valleys when I was growing up in the 1940s and 1950s, education was highly valued. It was seen as the escape from the only alternative – for the boys to going down the pit, and for the girls to secretarial or shop work. It was especially valued in my family because my father had had to fight so hard for his education and had finally 'made it'.

On hearing my decision, my father put his face close up to mine, wagged his finger at me, and said: 'Good gel, I don't care what you do afterwards, but you get your education first!'

At this point in my story, Rhodri Morgan bent closer and asked what was my maiden name. 'It was a dreadful name,' I replied, 'I was constantly teased as a child. It was Hickery – like the nursery rhyme.' 'Good God,' he said, 'you're Ernie Hickery's daughter aren't you! You're my third cousin.' He proceeded to describe a line between my maternal grandmother and his father, TJ Morgan, who had been Registrar of The University of Wales, and whom I vaguely remember my mother talking about as Uncle TJ. Given the 'everyone related to everyone else' characteristic of the Welsh, this was interesting but no big deal until he added: 'I remember it well because for months you ruined our family mealtimes. For months the conversation was always about what could "the family" do to help poor Ernie, who had this wilful, pigheaded daughter who was quite bright and he wanted her to go to university, but all she wanted to do was to be a bloody nurse!'

I did get the grades, and I did take up the place at University College London. Nursing just had to wait.

PART I: BEGINNINGS

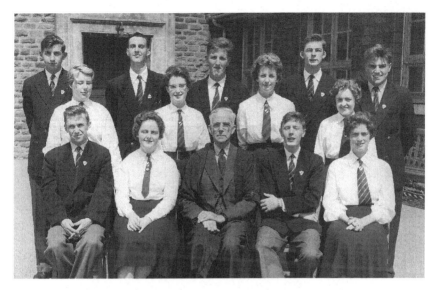

Upper sixth form, Pontywaun Grammar School 1958–9
(June is on the left of the middle row)

CHAPTER 1: ROOTS

I am proud of my Welsh heritage. I was brought up in the South Wales valleys and I am through and through the product of my roots. The values and ideals of the community in which I was raised – social justice, equality, rights and responsibilities, public service, standing up for what you believe in – still permeate everything I say and do today. We lived in Risca, just a few miles down the valley from Tredegar, the birthplace of 'Nye' Bevan and the NHS. I was not actually born in Wales, however; I was born in Sheffield, in 1941, as an accident of World War II. Not the usual sort of accident of war – it was just that my father was in a reserved occupation as a full-time trade union officer in the steel industry, and when war broke out he was relocated from Wales to Sheffield.

At the end of the war we moved back to Wales, and my father was appointed Divisional Officer for the British Iron and Steel Trade Association. Looking back I am very much my father's daughter. Born in 1904 in Gowerton, near Swansea, he left school at the age of 14 and went to work in the local steelworks, where he soon became involved in the developing trade union movement. He took every opportunity to 'get an education', using the evening classes provided by the Workers' Educational Association. In 1929, aged 25, he won a scholarship to Coleg Harlech, which had recently been established in association with the Workers' Educational Association. The scholarship lasted for a year, after which he went back to work in the steelworks. He worked there until in 1935 he won another scholarship, this time to Swansea University. Again, the scholarship was for 1 year only but, supported by the union, he combined study with work in the steelworks until finally, in 1939, he was able to graduate. It is undoubtedly this experience that explains his emphasis on the importance of education for his daughters – my younger sister Kay and me.

I remember my mother as the archetypal homemaker; when my father turned up at unusual times, often accompanied by members of some visiting delegation, she could always put a meal on the table. We children were expected to sit at the table on such occasions, and this was no doubt the beginning of my political education. Our mother made all our clothes, was an expert in crafts such as crochet and tatting, baked cakes, made brawn out of pigs' heads, and took care to pass on her skills to us. With the benefit of hindsight and my experience in nursing behind me, I think she was frustrated by the limitations of her role. She had begun a university education at Swansea, where she met my father, but was forced to give up when her younger brother got a Welsh Church Scholarship to Oxford.

Growing up in the South Wales valleys

I attended Risca Town Primary School and then, having passed the 11-plus exam, I started at Pontywaun Grammar School in September 1952. I remember that in our first geography class the teacher, whom we called Gertie, went round the class asking us what we wanted to be when we grew up. I said I wanted to be a lawyer like Rose Heilbron, who was at the time often in the newspapers as England's premier woman barrister; there was no mention at that time of any aspirations to be a nurse.

Yet the seed must have been there, because of all my teenage hobbies the only one that survived was my involvement with the St John Ambulance Brigade. I gave up Guides because camping with St John Ambulance (which had boys as well as girls) was much more fun! Most significantly, on Saturday mornings I caught the bus to Newport and went to St Woolos Hospital, where I 'worked' on the children's ward, helping with jobs such as feeding and changing babies and playing with the older children. I remained active in St John Ambulance until after I left Risca for university. Almost

60 years later I have picked it up again, this time becoming a member of the West Glamorgan Council and the Mumbles Division.

Whatever the debates nowadays about the merits or otherwise of grammar schools, Pontywaun Grammar School was the making of many Risca kids, including me. By today's standards it was a very small school, with an annual intake of 60 children and a total roll of about 300. Everybody – staff and pupils – knew everybody else in the school. We did not have the facilities or the range of subjects that larger schools have nowadays, but what we had was a good solid education. One teacher in particular was very special to me. This was John Herbert, who taught Latin. The choice of Classics for my university education was thus fixed. Mr Herbert became my personal counsellor as well as my teacher, and is probably the person who had the greatest influence on the most formative period of my growing up.

On only one occasion at Pontywaun did I not come top of my form: in Form 5 I dropped to second place (having come 16th in religious instruction). My school reports usually recorded 'Excellent', although sometimes with a barbed comment such as 'Does excellent work but is too talkative', and 'Excellent work – but a more co-operative attitude would make her achievement the more commendable'.

All pupils were allocated to one of four 'houses': Red, Blue, Yellow, and Green. I was in the Greens, and eventually became house captain. Each year there were two inter-house competitions: sports day in the summer and the eisteddfod in the spring. I was useless in the sports day, but I excelled in the eisteddfod. An eisteddfod is a Welsh tradition, a competitive festival of literature, music and performance; competitions include solo singing, choirs, instrumentalists, poetry reading, recitation and creative writing. I participated enthusiastically in the group events, such as the house choir and the 'choral speaking', and always did well in the creative writing competitions. I frequently won the poetry, short story and essay classes for my age group, with all of my winning pieces being published in the school magazine. Reading them now I see much of what I wrote as a teenager as pretentious rubbish, but I guess it must reflect how I felt at the time. One year I won the senior essay competition on the title 'The future', in which I set out a philosophy I have always maintained: 'There is one fact, however, that we must realise: our future is what we ourselves make it. It is the moral duty of every human being to strive to leave the world a better place than he found it.'

The big problem during my teen years, from my parents' point of view, was my boyfriend Maurice. Maurice left school at 15 and, along with many of his peers, joined his father down the pit. After the pit he went into the army. He reasoned that if he did not volunteer he would soon be called up anyway (our age group was the last to experience compulsory national service). He joined the parachute regiment, but it did not last long. I remember spending a night in the local police station where Maurice was held in the cells because he had gone AWOL: we had been in the cinema, and when the lights came up there were the military police, who marched him across the road to the police station. My parents were especially mortified because they were friendly with the local police inspector and his wife, who lived in the police station. Added to this, my sister and I were friendly with their two daughters.

The problem was that in my parents' eyes I was an academic high flyer destined for university and great things thereafter, while Maurice could barely read and write and had no interest in education. It was not a class thing – after all, my father had left school at 14 to work in the steelworks and was a keen socialist and trade union supporter. The issue was aspiration and education. Maurice had neither. I knew I was expected to go to university, and I wanted to go, but Maurice and I assumed I would then come back to Risca, find a job locally, marry, and live the same sort of life as his two older sisters, who were already married with children. That was not what my parents had planned for me.

Meanwhile I continued to excel at school. I sat the Oxford entrance exam and was called for interview. Some days later I received a letter asking me if I had considered reading Philosophy, Politics and Economics (or PPE). I had no idea what that was. Many years later, John Herbert wrote to me, saying: 'I suggested that she should decline.... I was so wrong. PPE would have been exactly the right pathway; I have had this on my conscience all my life. Did I stop June from being our first woman Prime Minister?'

I don't think so! Although I have always been interested in politics, I never saw myself as a member of parliament, much less a Maggie Thatcher. I was advised to go back to school for a third year in the sixth form (as most applicants did) and re-apply next year. In Pontywaun there was no special provision other than repeating the second year, and since all my peers would have left and I was already feeling that I had outgrown school, I was not prepared to do it. I chose University College London (UCL) instead and was offered a place to read Classics subject to success in my forthcoming A-level examinations. Only later did I come to understand the significance of my classical education, how it has shaped my ways of thinking and provided the seeds of my much later interest in concept analysis and nursing informatics.

At this point I had a major row with my father. I did not think I had done very well in my exams and announced that if I did not pass my A levels I was not willing to go back to school: I was going directly into nursing and I had already applied to and been accepted by the Royal Infirmary Cardiff. My father was furious. I can see him now, and have always remembered those words quoted in the Prologue: 'Good gel, I don't care what you do afterwards, but you get your education first!' (He always addressed me as 'good gel' when we were having a row.) The results came out, I passed, and my place at UCL was confirmed.

If I have one regret, it would be the pain and anxiety I caused my parents during my teenage years. I was certainly wilful and pig-headed. I had terrible rows with my father that often ended in tears – my mother's! Yet growing up during the 1950s in South Wales was much easier than growing up today. There were no drugs, there was no television, no social networking. The 'pop scene' was Radio Luxembourg at 11pm on Sunday evenings. The social scene was two Italian cafes, one at the top end of 'the road', and one at the bottom end that had a jukebox and served frothy coffee. Wednesday was early closing day and the pubs were shut on Sundays, except for the working men's club. People went to church or chapel at least once on Sunday, and after evening service the young people went on the 'monkey parade', which involved walking in small single-sex groups along the main road from one end of the village to the other, eyeing the groups of the opposite sex. The parameters were narrow and the boundaries were clear. Perhaps that is why I was so rebellious!

Expanding horizons

Going to university in London was a huge culture shock. At Pontywaun I had been a big fish in a little pond; at UCL I was a very little fish in a very big pond, and it was a struggle to swim. At Pontywaun I had always been top of the class; in the Classics Department at UCL I was usually at the bottom.

Early in our first term my tutor asked me to investigate a subject of my own choosing, and I chose early Roman comedy. I spent a long time in the huge College library, which was bigger than any library I had seen before and had a wonderful 'book smell' that I still remember and love. I was quite proud of what I produced, but was quite taken aback when we discussed it in my tutorial and my tutor said that I was now more knowledgeable about the subject than he was (which I am sure was not true) and I should go back to the library and expand what I had written as my assignment for my next tutorial. It was a way of teaching and learning that I have held on to throughout my career, and quite different from what I later experienced in nursing education.

In the first year I was allocated a place at Canterbury Hall in Cavendish Square, a hall of residence for women from all the colleges of London University. This provided me with my first experience of people from other countries and other cultures. I had my first taste of curry in the rather seedy Indian restaurant round the corner from the Hall. I became more and more interested in the world outside the UK.

Despite the vibrant culture and supportive tutor, I found my first months in London difficult. I think this was the reason that that half way through my first term I got engaged to Maurice. Somehow I felt that an engagement ring gave me some kind of status among my colleagues that made up for my lack of academic success. My parents, of course, were in despair. At the end of my first year I booked myself and Maurice on a holiday to Greece organised by the United Nations Students Association, whose chairman that year was a Greek called Kostas Kleanthous. I was of course thrilled to see all the antiquities that I knew from my academic studies, but Maurice did not seem interested in anything or happy in the company of the group. With hindsight I think I was already beginning to realise how much I had changed since leaving Risca; I could see that the world was a far bigger place than I had ever imagined, and that Maurice just did not fit with it.

At the end of my first year, in despair at my lack of academic success, I suggested to my personal tutor, Dr Jack Kells, that perhaps I should leave before I was pushed. He laughed and said that if the department had made a mistake in accepting me as a student they would stand by their mistake. He thought I would probably not get a first but was perfectly capable of getting an upper two. He told me I should stop worrying and start to enjoy myself. So I did.

I was very lucky in getting a place in Canterbury Hall in the second year as places were in short supply and first-year and overseas students were given priority. I stood for election as Hall President and came second in the poll, so I became Vice-President, which guaranteed me a place for my third year. I became Secretary of the Classics Society, which was the Department's 'social arm'. I started going to the students' union meetings. My academic performance improved, although alpha marks remained elusive.

By the beginning of my third year I knew I could not marry Maurice and go back to live in Risca. About a month into term I went home for the weekend, and when we went for a walk I told Maurice that I could not go through with it: as soon as I finished university I was going into nursing.

In the middle of the night on our doorstop he shot himself using a double-barrelled shotgun. He was admitted to the Royal Gwent Hospital, and he survived. Not only was attempted suicide at this time a criminal offence, but in a community like Risca it was a major scandal. I had to get back to London. If I was going to start a new life I had better start it immediately.

I tried to get on with university life but I had terrible nightmares and flashbacks. I could not concentrate on anything. Nowadays I suppose we would call it post-traumatic stress disorder. I knew that I needed to talk about it, but I did not know who to talk to. I thought about who among my university friends might be able to help. The first two people I thought of were away for the weekend, but the third – Roger Clark – was in.

Every year the whole Classics Department (staff and students, about 30 of us in all) went away for a residential weekend somewhere, where we were able to get to know one another and integrate the new intake of students. Roger and I had worked together on the organisation of that year's event, so when I arrived on his doorstep Roger thought that it was something to do with Classics Society business. 'No,' I said, 'I just need somebody to talk to about something. I don't need you to do anything, I just need to be able to pour it all out.' He looked at me and walked across the room. 'I'll put the kettle on,' he said.

One day Roger said: 'I think you are sufficiently rehabilitated by now, and the Hall Ball is coming up. I can get free tickets because I'm on the committee. Would you like to go?' In those days, university balls were grand occasions. The favourite venue was the Royal Festival Hall, full evening dress was required, and the event started at 11pm and ended at 5am with breakfast and a walk home through the Covent Garden flower market. That year we went to three.

At Christmas a problem arose. I wanted to spend the minimum possible time in Risca. To this end, I arranged to stay in Canterbury Hall along with the overseas students but there was a gap of 3 days when Hall was closed. 'Well you'd better come and stay with us in Sevenoaks,' said Roger. 'We've plenty of space and I'm sure my parents wouldn't mind.' Years later my (future) in-laws said that of course they 'knew', but I can honestly say that at that time the thought had never entered my head. I was in no fit state for a new relationship. In fact, having decided to start nursing as soon as I graduated, I assumed that I would be less and less available and Roger would soon find someone else.

When finals arrived the stress brought back all the nightmares and the flashbacks. I was convinced I had failed, and was ashamed that I would be letting everyone at home down. My father and Mr Herbert were sure I was going to get a first, and nothing I could say could persuade them otherwise.

I got alphas for my four special subjects (pre-Socratic philosophy, Plato, Aristotle, and Roman comedy) and for my general essay paper, but barely passed the language papers. I totally failed the Latin prose. Dr Handley, my personal tutor, sent a card that said: 'Can I join in and say how very pleased I am to hear by the grapevine of some most distinguished results in some of the papers which wiped out the trouble with the Latin prose and left you sailing to a clear and well-deserved result overall. Many congratulations and good wishes.' Perhaps I would have done better if I had read Philosophy rather than Classics. We shall never know. Now that I have sat on a great many examination boards, I can well understand the dilemma that the board must have had over such an erratic student.

In October I started my nursing studies. Contrary to my expectations, Roger and I did not drift apart; we stayed close, and a year later we got engaged. In those days student nurses who got married were required to leave, so we planned for a wedding in July 1966 after I qualified. Meanwhile my younger sister also got engaged and planned a wedding just 3 weeks after ours. That provided us with a good reason for our wedding not to be in Risca. Even though Maurice was now married with two children, I still feared his shadow. We decided it would be at Roger's home in Sevenoaks. As a mother of four boys but no daughter, Roger's mum, Peggy, was delighted.

Meanwhile Roger had graduated and had started work in the Registrar's department at Reading University. All University staff members were allocated to a hall of residence as members of the senior common room, and several lived in. In 1965 there was a sudden expansion in student numbers, and to provide extra accommodation the University opened up, at very short notice, two adjacent 'student houses' in Craven Road that had recently been closed pending the building of a new maternity unit for the hospital next door. Roger was asked to take over as stand-in warden of what became known as 'Craven Palace'. Three months later I arrived in Reading to begin my midwifery training, living in the nurse's home but spending all of my off-duty time with Roger in Craven Palace. Roger loved his year as warden, and so was delighted when he was asked to take up a similar position at another student house that was being refurbished as an annexe to the newly-built Windsor Hall. Foxhill House was scheduled to open in October 1966, and it had a flat for a member of staff. This was exactly the time when we would be looking for accommodation after our wedding in July.

We were married on 23 July 1966 at the little church of St Peter and St Paul in Seal. It was a lovely wedding. We went back to work on Monday, delaying our honeymoon by a week because at that time the cheap student flights to Athens went only on Saturdays. The builders were already in our flat at Foxhill; we lasted in the flat until Thursday, when the toilets were closed down, and then went 'home to Mum' until we could leave for Greece.

We had a wonderful honeymoon. It was not the kind of luxury package that a couple would have today. With our rucksacks on our backs we arrived in Athens in the afternoon and booked into the cheapest hotel we could find; it was not until 3 o'clock the next morning that we found we had chosen the street where the meat market was held. We decided to get out of Athens as soon as possible and head for Crete but there were two things we needed to do before we left. The first was to get our student cards, which would give us free admission to all the antiquities and museums. This was important not only for obvious 'cultural' reasons, but also because the museums were the only places with clean lavatories and a washbasin! The second was to go to the local hospital to sell a pint of blood. The trick, known to all students, was to sell a pint of blood at the beginning of the holiday, which would provide enough money to live on for a week or so, and then sell another pint on the last day, when getting home would enable recovery. In the villages we slept on the flat roofs of the village tavernas, where the deal was a place on the roof in exchange for eating at their taverna. To this day the only phrase of modern Greek that I can remember is: 'Please can we sleep on your roof?' In Malia we slept on the beach, and I remember waking at dawn to the heavenly scent of the lilies that were portrayed on the murals and pottery that we saw in Knossos. I can still smell them now.

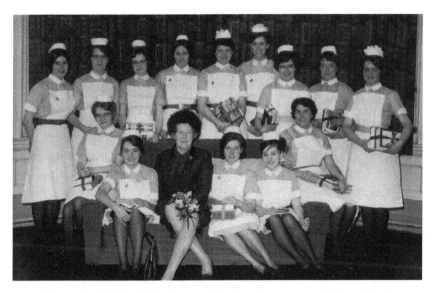

Prizegiving UCH 1966 (June is in the back row, second from right)

CHAPTER 2: INTO NURSING

I wanted so much to be a nurse. My parents were not pleased and my friends thought I was mad. I had just completed a university degree in Classics at University College London (UCL). My tutor asked me why I didn't just do a PhD on Hippocrates. My grandma, who tried to be kind, said: 'Never mind love, all that Latin won't be wasted – you'll be able to read the prescriptions. And you might find a nice doctor to marry.' Whatever the reasons, I know only that I wanted to be a nurse and with an intensity that kept me going through everything, even when the rational part of me told me that I must be mad. This passion has kept me in nursing for more than 50 years.

After my 3 years as an undergraduate in London I knew I wanted to remain in London. This was a challenge, as I had heard that getting into a London teaching hospital was like getting into Eton – you had to put your name down almost at birth. I thought that perhaps University College Hospital (UCH) would take me because of my recent connection with UCL, so I applied there and nowhere else, and was soon asked to attend an interview. Matron Helen Downton was a formidable woman – 7 feet tall (or so it seemed), very angular, and with enormous hands and feet. She wore a beautifully tailored navy blue dress and a frilly white cap of a style unique to herself. She grilled me for half an hour about why I wanted to be a nurse and warned me that it would be very hard work. In due course I received a letter accepting my application and asking me to present myself at the Rockefeller Nurses' Home in Gordon Street, WC1, on Sunday 22 September 1962.

The first year

I crossed Gower Street from UCL to UCH. Gower Street is not a very wide road, but it was like stepping across a time warp. I am reminded of the television series *Goodnight Sweetheart*, where Nicholas Lyndhurst played Gary Sparrow, who discovers that by walking through a wall he can travel between 1990s London and the London of World War II. It was just like that. I remember thinking as I stood on the doorstep 'What the hell have I let myself in for?' The building is still there, with 'NURSES HOME' carved into the concrete archway over the door, although it has long ceased to be used for that purpose.

As a student nurse, 'living in' in the Rockefeller Nurses' Home was compulsory. We each had a little white room containing an iron bedstead with starched white sheets and a white bedspread, a small table with a chair and a desk lamp, a chest of drawers, a wardrobe and a washbasin. My little room was like a thousand other rooms in nurses' homes all over the world at that time. Indeed, I stayed in one just like it at the University of Iowa School of Nursing some 25 years later. Every moveable item – bed linen, towels, china, even the (hard and shiny) toilet paper, was stamped 'Property of University College Hospital'. At the end of the corridor there were a couple of bathrooms, the toilets and a kitchen, the latter being the place where we assembled to gossip about people's love lives and what had happened on the ward. On the first floor was Home Sister's office, to which we had to report if ever we were sick or needed a light bulb.

Down on the ground floor was the dining room for students and staff nurses – sisters and more senior nurses had a separate dining room in a different nurses' home in what is now the Grafton Hotel on Tottenham Court Road – and a large room which was properly called the lounge, but was known to everyone as the 'passion parlour' because it was the only place in the building where we were allowed to take men. It had several sofas and big armchairs and nice soft carpet, the curtains were always tightly drawn, and the lights were never on. There was also a library, which was a small panelled room with glass-fronted bookcases. This was kept locked, but the key was available on request from Sister Tutor. Finally, there was a large classroom with individual desks with inkwells similar to those I had used during the 1940s and 50s at school. In the basement there were the 'practical rooms', that is, classrooms whose walls were lined with posters showing various views of the human body and glass cases containing body organs pickled in formalin. These rooms were fitted out with beds and other equipment on which we would practice our nursing skills.

This was the swinging 60s, and the Beatles were top of the hit parade, but it was also the time when the Minister of Health, Enoch Powell, stood on a platform to justify rejecting the latest nurses' pay claim on the grounds that nurses enjoyed the special perk of enhanced marriage prospects! Nursing students had to be in by 10 o'clock, but round the back in the mews there was a sash window that was carefully kept ajar for latecomers. The alternative was the underground corridors that connected all parts of UCH to the Nurses' Home, but that required running the gauntlet of Night Sister's rounds. Our doors did have a key, but the dragon-like Home Sister had a master key, and would descend without warning, ostensibly to check that we had made our beds correctly and damp-dusted all surfaces, but more likely to check that there was no evidence of unauthorised occupation – especially male. Of course we were all women. There were no male nurses except in psychiatric hospitals, which were regarded as rather nasty places.

Each cohort of new students was numbered consecutively. I was part of set 156. There were 50 of us in my set, which was the largest set that UCH had ever had. We were all young, female, single (marriage was not allowed), and mostly straight out of school. The London teaching hospitals at that time took the 'crème de la crème', often from medical families, often from private schools.

The course was organised so that each set did everything together: we lived together, went onto night duty together (for 3 months each year), and went on holiday together. The sets formed a strict social hierarchy. You simply did not sit in the same place in the dining room as the set above you, and you did not talk to anyone in the set below you, except to boss them around when you were on the ward and in charge. In those days, and right up to the mid-1990s, students were the hospital's main workforce. We were there to do the work, with a bit of learning thrown in for a couple of weeks a year when we 'went into block', i.e. came off the wards into the School of Nursing for a couple of weeks of lectures. It sounds awful, but in fact the set was a huge source of mutual support.

Initiation

On our first morning at Rockefeller Nurses' Home we assembled in the classroom for the preliminary training school (PTS). This was the period of 12 weeks' theoretical and practical instruction we would receive before being 'released' into 'real' nursing on the wards. First, however, there were administrative tasks to complete. We were each given an appointment to go to the sewing room, where we were individually measured for our grey-and-white striped dresses (length 14 inches from the floor), and issued with white starched collars and frilled cotton cuffs, eight starched aprons, and four flat starched semicircles of cotton material that we would be taught to manipulate into our nurses' caps. These items would be sent weekly to the laundry, from where they would return as stiff as cardboard and be placed as a parcel in our rooms. We were also issued with our beautiful grey woollen, red-fabric-lined capes. We were never allowed to wear our uniforms outside the Hospital, except much later when we were allowed to 'live out', when we could wear our dresses (not caps or aprons) under the regulation navy blue Burberry mac. I was so proud of my uniform. I appreciate that the modern scrubs that most nurses now wear are more practical and more hygienic, but I regret its passing.

We spent a whole morning learning how to fold our caps. Our tutors were Sister Clare and Sister Wilmott, and they had an assistant called Staff Nurse Lovegrove, whose claim to fame was that, against all the regulations, she made her cap into a tiny concoction that perched on top of her hair like a butterfly. We learnt anatomy and physiology with bits of bones and plastic models. The tutors' teaching aids were primitive. I shall never forget Sister Clare standing in the front of the class with her arms spread saying: 'I am a uterus and these are my fallopian tubes.' I always wanted to learn more, and I found the illustrations in the physiology textbooks frustrating, so I persuaded a medical student with whom I had become friendly to smuggle me in with him to observe a post mortem. Unfortunately I could not keep my mouth shut about what I had seen, so the tutors found out and I was carpeted – the first of many occasions – for 'going beyond my business as a nurse'.

We also learnt how to make beds with hospital corners, how to make a kaolin poultice, how to make egg custard and beef tea, how to lay up the trolley for numerous technical procedures having boiled up the forceps, etc in the steriliser (no disposables in those days), how to open a bottle of medicine with your little finger, how to damp dust and why it is important, and how to bandage (a skill that I have always found useful). We were also told things like: 'Never give anyone a cold bedpan. Run it under the hot water tap and be careful to dry it.' At the time bedpans were made of stainless steel and one of the jobs on our first ward was to polish them to keep them shining. We even learned how to apply leeches and do cupping, although we were told that these treatments were 'not used much nowadays'.

In the fifth week of our training we visited the wards where we would start work after PTS was finished. We assembled at the door of the School of Nursing and, in a long crocodile with Sister Tutor at our head, we marched through the hospital leaving a forlorn and frightened figure at the door of each ward en route. On the third floor it was my turn. I pushed the swing door and found myself in ward 32, a 'mixed' ward divided into three small ones and a number of single rooms. At that time it was the only ward in UCH structured in this way – all the others were large 'Nightingale' wards – so it took a mixture of patients, including children. There was not a nurse in sight except for the ward sister writing at a desk. She looked up briefly and said: 'Oh, er, I'll be with you in a moment, but would you go and help the physio with Mr Jenkins [not his real name] for a minute. Bed 5, over there.' She indicated a curtained bed in the first small ward. I crept through the gap in the curtains to find a girl in a white coat with her back to me turning back the counterpane. 'Oh good,' she said without looking back, 'hold that please.' She handed me a plastic bag full of yellow liquid. I just had time to register that the grey face on the pillow was that of an elderly man before she flung back the sheet. The man was wearing only a pyjama jacket, there was a tube coming out of his nose, another out of his penis attached to the bag I was holding, and a colostomy to which another bag was attached.

I was 21 years old, but I had never seen a naked man before. If I looked as if I was going to be sick, the physiotherapist was much too busy to notice. She lifted the man's head and shoulders forward from the pillow and swung his legs over the side of the bed. She was watching his face all the time. 'Put his slippers on,' she said. She did not look at me. I bent down and did as she commanded, leaving the bag, which I was still clutching, on the bed. Together we lifted him to his feet. I was terrified that he would fall. My hands and feet seemed not to belong to me. 'Thanks Nurse,' she said, 'I can manage now.' She smiled briefly in dismissal. Throughout the procedure the man had not uttered a sound nor looked at either of us. I crept back through the gap in the curtains. There was still not a nurse in sight. Even the ward sister had vanished. I did not see her again. Indeed I visited the ward twice more before I saw her a second time. The rest of the afternoon passed in a sort of haze. I remember pushing a trolley and pouring out cups of tea, and then it was time to go off duty.

On my second visit to the ward, a week after the first, there was another man in Mr Jenkins' bed. No-one commented on the fact. I could not make myself ask what had happened to Mr Jenkins. I blinked at the new face and tried to forget that there had ever been another there before. I could not talk about the feelings with which I could not cope. I would not even admit to myself that the experience had been a shock. In any case there was no-one I could talk to about it. I was afraid my friends would laugh. I told myself that I was just naive; after all, hospitals were there for people who were very ill, and of course people died, and I had better get used to it. After all, it was my own decision to be a nurse and that was what nursing was all about. I put the whole incident firmly to the back of my mind. I was already learning to build the protective shell identified by Isobel Menzies' research as the 'mental defence mechanisms' that make some nurses seem hard and lacking in compassion.

At the end of PTS we put on a show for our teachers. We did sketches and parodies of popular songs. I remember in particular the one sung to the tune of My Bonnie lies Over the Ocean. Each verse related to one of the tutors or one of us or some aspect of our PTS experience. The final chorus went:

'The biggest, the baddest, the wildest,
Some say we're just living for kicks,
But one day you'll see 'cos we'll prove it,
That the best set was set 156.'

That turned out to be prophetic. Among several other achievements, set 156 produced three of the first professors of nursing: Professor Dame Jill Macleod Clark (then June Gibbs), Professor Jean Macintosh (then Jean Cresswell), and myself.

Introduction to nursing politics

My initiation into nursing politics came early. Within my first month of training I was elected the 'Set Rep' on the hospital student committee, then was elected first to the Council and then to the Chair of the National Student Nurses Association (SNA). In November 1963 I represented the SNA at the annual meeting of the National Union of Students – the first student nurse ever to attend. A motion that condemned 'the archaic principles governing the lives of student nurses' was passed unanimously, and in *The Guardian* I was quoted as saying: 'This country does not expect the education of its children to be in the hands of student teachers; an engineering works does not run on the labour of apprentices; but 74% of the labour of nursing the sick in hospitals is provided by student nurses.' The headline, not the first or the last of its kind, was 'Student nurses – just a cheap pair of hands'. When I became Chair of the SNA, among the letters of congratulation was one from the National Union of Students Publicity Officer, which said: 'It has been very obvious to many people that your militancy has helped student nurses considerably.' It was not, however, very obvious to me, and certainly not to Matron!

One of my earliest initiatives in the hospital was to organise a debate on the motion that 'This house believes that the nurse is but the doctor's handmaiden'. The main proposer and opposer were a doctor and a ward sister who were widely rumoured to be in a relationship. UCH was always alive with such rumours about doctor–nurse romances, but the idea undoubtedly added spice to the occasion. The passion parlour, where the meeting was held, was packed out, and the motion was overwhelmingly defeated.

In June 1965 I represented British students at the 13th International Council of Nurses (ICN) Quadrennial Congress in Frankfurt. Although at this time the ICN did not recognise students as members, about 100 students from 18 countries attended and we held two meetings for students. We shared information about student associations in the various countries, and elected a student committee (of which I was a member), with a commitment to press for recognition within the ICN and to make arrangements for the next Congress, which was due to be held in 1969.

The 1965 ICN Congress ignited an interest in nursing in other countries that has persisted throughout my nursing career. One of the earliest spin-offs was the opportunity for a 3-week exchange visit to my opposite number in Sweden, and a placement at the Södersjukhuset Hospital in Stockholm.

It was also the first occasion on which I quite unexpectedly experienced a standing ovation. It came during the question time following a plenary presentation about the future of nursing education. I rose to my feet to point out that student nurses were always eager to learn but were not always so eager to be taught – a point that did not seem at all strange to me but appeared to be a novel thought for the rest of the audience.

At national level, our SNA Council came to be known as 'the Ginger Group' because we complained about what we saw as the patronising attitude of the Royal College of Nursing (RCN), who at that time provided our leadership and funding. (Later I was to lead the negotiations that eventually brought the SNA into the RCN as the 'Student Section'.) We also negotiated with Peggy Nuttall, editor of the *Nursing Times*, to have a special page for students in the magazine that was to be written by us. This initiative can probably now be identified as the beginning of my writing career.

And so started my long career in nursing politics. I am still at it. Current pay struggles and ballots about industrial action are not new; during the 70s and 80s, when the struggle was far more vitriolic than it is now, we marched, we waved banners, and we besieged the Houses of Parliament. It is not allowed now, but I remember marching from RCN Headquarters to Trafalgar Square and then standing up high by the lions shouting into a megaphone. My speech was immediately followed by an equally rousing speech by Michael Foot. We held a silent vigil for 3 days in the Houses of Parliament – working in shifts we kept a nurse in uniform 24 hours a day in the front row of the public gallery.

Into 'real' nursing

After 3 months in PTS we were let loose on the wards. At the time this was known as ward allocation, not clinical placements, and we did 12 weeks in each one before moving onto the next. I guess everyone remembers their first day on the wards and I remember that day vividly. Although I had visited the ward several times during PTS, this was 'the real thing'. I was sent to help Staff Nurse (we were never addressed by our first names) who was doing the drug round. All the bottles of pills were carefully laid out on a bed-table, which we pushed from bed to bed. Staff Nurse checked each chart, reminded me of the mantra that we all learnt to say ('Right patient, right drug, right dose, right route, right time.'), put the pills in a little pot, and told me to give it to the man in Bed 1. By the fourth patient I reminded myself that I was supposed to be learning something, so I asked whether she could tell me what the pills were and why we were giving them to the patient. She drew herself up over her blue belt (different coloured belts indicated how senior you were) and said: 'Nurse Hickery, you are not here to ask questions; you are here to do the work. Please get on with it.' Now of course I realise that she probably did not know the answer, but no nurse would ever admit this, and certainly not to a junior.

It was on another drug round on the same ward that I made my first drug error. It was salbutamol, a drug prescribed to help people with respiratory disorders to breathe more easily. In those days we used to give salbutamol per rectum as suppositories. I put the dish containing the two suppositories on the patient's locker and went to get the special tray with the gloves and the lubricant from the utility room. When I got back to the patient the dish was empty and the suppositories were gone – he had eaten them! It was the early morning round and we were desperately busy because there was trouble if everything was not done before Sister came on duty, but Night Sister, to whom I had to report it, required that I took and recorded his pulse every 15 minutes until the end of the shift. She was making sure that I would not forget or repeat my mistake.

I remember my first death, as I guess every nurse does. It was during the last great London smog, and the male medical section of the ward was full of gasping and coughing old men. They could hardly breathe, and the drugs and oxygen equipment that we could offer were, by today's standards, primitive. I spent a lot of time looking after a wizened little man who had lung cancer and it was clear that he was going to die. He was a heavy smoker and obviously malnourished; he lived in the poor area of London from which many of our patients came. I had the real honour of keeping him comfortable, feeding him, washing him, and giving him clean sheets when he was incontinent. He never said much, but it was a very special relationship, and it saddens me terribly that today's wards are so frantic that nurses rarely get time for that kind of thing. I was there when he died, and had the great privilege of being responsible for his 'last offices'. That meant washing him and laying him out, but also putting together his property for his relatives to collect – except that it seemed he had no relatives. He only ever had one visitor, a woman who came every Friday, who I assumed was his wife. It was only when I was putting together the pathetic little bag of his possessions after he had died that I found his rent book and realised that it was his landlady who came every week to collect the rent. She was the only person who cared enough to visit him, and that for the wrong reason. I think that was the day when I first knew I wanted to be a community nurse, because I wanted to work with people and their families in the real world, and not in the hothouse of a hospital.

I cannot understand why among some of today's nurses what is called 'basic nursing care' is seen as something to be delegated to less qualified mortals, such as healthcare assistants, nor why graduate nurses are accused of being 'too posh to wash and too clever to care'. For me, such tasks as bathing or feeding a seriously ill patient demand the greatest level of skill and bring the greatest job satisfaction. I thought about this a lot when, several years later, my own father was dying. At 78 he had enjoyed rude health all his life and had had little to do with doctors or hospitals until the 'indigestion' with which he had lived for some time suddenly became considerably worse. He was admitted to our local hospital for an operation to relieve the obstruction, which turned out to be a carcinoma of the pancreas. The surgeon did his job, and did it well, but we all knew the implications of the diagnosis. For the remaining 4 months of his life 'making the best of today' became our shared goal. The miracles of high-tech medicine and the skill of the surgeon gave him that extra time, and the wonders of the pharmaceutical industry ensured that they were relatively pain free. The things that contributed most to 'making the best of today', however, were knowing how to choose food that not only contained the nutrients necessary to encourage healing but would be acceptable in the absence of any appetite or sense of taste, finding a comfortable position in which to sleep (not easy when it involves changing the habits of a lifetime), finding new activities compatible with increasing weakness, giving him a warm bath and a shave, and the opportunity to talk through feelings – of anger, bitterness, loneliness, past happiness, or even hopes for the future. As a daughter I was never more grateful for my training as a nurse, nor for the ability to call on the skills of other nursing colleagues. The challenge of caring for my father stretched my nursing knowledge and skills to the limit.

Although they may appear to be no more than common sense, I believe that care skills are far more complex and demanding than many of the more technical and mechanical skills of medicine. When the final phase came, it was those skills for which both my father and I were most grateful. I was able to assist him in maintaining his dignity, self-determination and individuality until he died. When it became obvious that he had only a few days to live, my sister came to stay. The flexibility afforded by my job as a part-time health visitor meant I was able to keep working and come back to him at intervals during the day while she stayed with him all the time. On one occasion when I came back I found him lying in an obviously uncomfortable position, and I upbraided my sister about it. She cared about him just as much as I did, but she said that she had felt helpless because she did not know how to move him and was afraid that if she tried it would make things worse. I was able to lift him into a more comfortable position, wash his face and hands, and re-arrange his pillows using those 'basic' skills that I had learnt all those years ago. As I finished he whispered: 'Good gel, I was against you going into nursing, but I'm glad now that you did.'

There were other patients too who stick in the memory. One was a young man who was dying of Hodgkin disease, which was incurable in those days, and who was in constant pain. He was prescribed morphine 4-hourly, but however bad the pain we were not allowed to give him his injection a moment before the appointed time. Another was a heroin addict who had written a book about his 'recovery' from addiction, only to relapse later. He too was prescribed medication (heroin) in strictly controlled doses at strictly controlled times, and he cried like a baby for half an hour before his next dose could be given. Expert pain management and the good palliative care systems developed by Dr Cicely Saunders and others would not allow such suffering nowadays.

I also remember the 8-year-old child who was admitted with serious burns after standing too near an unguarded fire. In those days, people with extensive burns rarely survived. She had burns to her head, arms, chest, abdomen, and legs. There were no specialist burns units, but on the plus side our ward had individual cubicles and a skilled consultant plastic surgeon. Mr Matthews had learnt his skills under the supervision of the famous Dr Archie McIndoe, the plastic surgeon who had developed new techniques and achieved miracles for young fighter pilots badly burned during World War II. We nursed the girl on a net hammock suspended from a wooden frame fitted over the bed, and observed very strict barrier nursing procedures to prevent the burns becoming infected. This meant that before entering her cubicle we put on white gowns and masks and caps, which covered us completely except our eyes, rather like the Muslim burkha. One day when I was in her cubicle she said: 'This is a funny place. All bricks. But I like you because you've got nice eyes.' I realised that since she could not move except to turn her head to the right, the only things she could see were the brick wall outside her window and the eyes of the nurses who came to her. The good news was that she did survive – scarred and in need of extensive plastic surgery – but I was proud to have been part of the team who nursed her, and grateful for the way she made me think.

There were good times too. Christmas was wonderful. About a week before 25 December we used to wear our uniforms to Covent Garden, which was then a fruit and vegetable market, and beg for fruit and flowers for the wards' Christmas celebrations. The night nurses spent hours making decorations and we had a competition for the best decorated ward. (There were no health and safety restrictions in those days.) We used to keep one side room as a 'retreat' for staff, where we had all sorts of goodies that people had given us. Very few people had Christmas off. I liked to work the early shift on Christmas Eve, so that I could join in when we walked the wards carrying lanterns and singing carols, our red-lined capes turned inside out. On Christmas Day I would work a late shift so that I could go on duty early and join the festivities, with the consultant surgeon carving the turkey for lunch. Boxing Day would be my half day, followed by my day off so I was able to go home to my family.

I cannot say that I enjoyed my experience on that first ward, but I am glad I experienced it. I spent many hours in the sluice room ferociously polishing bedpans, and sometimes shedding a few tears. My experience made me angry, and determined to put right some of the things I was seeing. I was angry for the patients but also for the nurses, and especially for us students. And I said so, which was not a popular thing to do. In discussing my report at the end of my time on ward 32, the sister said that she did not think I would last a year. It gave me a great kick some years later when we met again in quite different circumstances to be able to say that not only had I completed my training, but that I was successfully building my nursing career.

Junior nights

My second ward, and my first night duty, was the post-natal ward in the maternity unit. A midwife had charge of the ward, and there was a senior student nurse who enjoyed the opportunity to boss me about. As she was in her third year, she was allowed to 'live out' and her main occupation seemed to be collecting any milk that had gone sour and putting it in a muslin napkin to drain over the kitchen sink to make cheese. I was the junior. On arrival on duty my first job was to collect all the empty feeding bottles, wash them in the big sink in the ward kitchen, and then put them to boil into a huge fish kettle on the gas stove. Thereafter it was to provide bedpans when required, as mothers were not encouraged to get up, and produce a constant supply of cups of tea for everyone. The most important job was to cook breakfast for the midwife at 4 am. At 6 am the fish kettle was called into service again to boil 30 eggs in a muslin napkin. Over time I perfected the technique for ensuring that they all came out soft-boiled. The babies did not stay with their mothers overnight; they slept together in the nursery, while those who cried were put separately into the linen room to prevent them waking the others. It was a lovely, if misguided, privilege to feed a baby while the mother slept.

One night I went to comfort a mother who was crying into her pillow. I knew that she was a 'grand multip', having just given birth to her seventh baby. I asked her why she was crying, and in reply she sobbed: 'Oh nurse, will I fall while I'm nursing him?' To my everlasting shame I did not understand what she was saying, and in my naivety I tried to reassure her that when she got home she would soon recover her old confidence. It was only later, during my health visitor training, that I came to realise how for women such as this one, at a time when birth control was not part of the NHS and charitable clinics were few and far between, another pregnancy was an absolute disaster. In a side room of the same ward at the same time we were nursing a seriously ill young girl suffering from septicaemia as the result of a botched illegal abortion.

Challenging the status quo

I was never a very good student. I always got good marks in the examinations, but I was never going to get the gold medal that was given to the 'best nurse' in each set. I was always in trouble. The trouble was that I would ask questions, and I would challenge things that had been around and unchallenged for 100 years. In particular I challenged the fact that student nurses were seen as employees and not as students. The struggle for 'student status' was not won until Project 2000 was implemented at the beginning of the 1990s, and there are still some who advocate a return to the old 'apprenticeship model'.

I was seen as a troublemaker, even to the extent that some sisters refused to have me on their wards. My reputation as 'The Graduate' (long before the Dustin Hoffman film) went before me. Looking back I can see that my position in the SNA and the RCN protected me at this time, and I was supported by wonderful mentors such as Baroness Jean McFarlane and other RCN leaders of the day. Much of my aggression could be directed at national level without detriment to the reputation of the hospital. At that time Sister Mary Whittow, a member of the RCN Council, ran what everyone agreed was probably the best ward in UCH: ward 44, which was the professorial medical unit. By the end of my first year my clinical experience had been entirely in specialist areas, as in those days clinical placements were allocated on the basis of a hospital's workforce needs and not the student's learning needs. I was too junior to participate in the technical procedures, so my role was limited to cleaning bedpans and making tea, and I felt I had had no opportunity to learn about or to do 'real' nursing. I went to see Matron and asked for a placement on ward 44 and luckily she agreed. My placement there was the best of my whole student experience. What I did not know until years later was that every time I was in trouble and in danger of being sacked, Mary Whittow would go to Matron and plead my case. Amid present-day debates about the lack of 'clinical leadership' at the ward level, Mary Whittow was a shining example of what a ward sister should be.

At the beginning of my second year I found myself in trouble because I had responded to an article in the medical students' magazine that criticised the lack of clinical teaching that medical students received. I pointed out that student nurses received even less, and were more vulnerable because they were an integral part of the workforce carrying direct responsibility for patient care. I was summoned to Matron's office and informed in no uncertain terms that the hospital existed for the benefit of patients and not of the nurses: Matron could only conclude that I 'had no ideals of service'. I retreated to my little white room in the nurses' home and cried. The next day in the ward, however, the certain knowledge that such skill as I had acquired had enabled me to make just one old lady just a little bit more comfortable – I could see it written on her face – was enough to set me sailing on a cloud of happiness. Moreover, I reasoned, Matron was just plain wrong.

Psychiatric placement

My second year included the placement that has probably had the greatest influence on my thinking as a nurse: 12 weeks at Friern Hospital in North London. Friern Hospital, formerly called the Colney Hatch Lunatic Asylum, was one of the ring of large psychiatric hospitals the Victorians had built around the edges of London to house the mentally ill detritus of the capital.

Friern Hospital itself was enormous. At the time it housed almost 2000 patients. Around a central dome above the main entrance hall were two wings: the 'male side' and the 'female side'. The corridor from one end to the other was almost half a mile long and said to be the longest in Europe. On the male side, male nurses nursed male patients, and on the female side, female nurses nursed female patients. The sexes (patients and nurses) rarely met, except in the newly-developing therapeutic departments, which consisted of occupational therapy – then called 'industrial therapy' – or in 'accidental' encounters in the hospital grounds. The hospital was situated in large grounds, which included the farm and kitchen garden that provided food for the hospital and work for its inmates. The whole place was enclosed within a high wall. It was one of the hospitals described in Barbara Robb's seminal attack on the iniquities of such institutions in *Sans Everything*, and exactly as described in Goffman's book *Asylums*. My experience there was shocking.

The first ward, where we worked for 4 weeks, was an acute admission ward for psychotic patients, mostly suffering from schizophrenia. It was the first time I had witnessed psychotic behaviour or met patients suffering from visual hallucinations or obvious delusions. Violent behaviour was not uncommon; I remember the young woman who barred herself into the washroom, broke all the windows and tore two washbasins from the wall before she was restrained. The ward was locked, so we carried a bunch of keys that allowed the nurses but not the patients to come and go. The smell of paraldehyde, given as a sedative or to stop seizures, permeated the ward. Most patients were given large doses of chlorpromazine (Largactil) or trifluoperazine (Stelazine), given in syrup form because that was the best way of ensuring that it was swallowed. For night sedation most patients received large doses of chloral hydrate, also in syrup form. Medication management was very different from my experience in the general hospital: here the patients would line up at the door of the treatment room to receive their medication, usually on a spoon from a large bottle shared by all.

The other preferred form of treatment, especially for patients suffering from severe depression, was electroconvulsive therapy (ECT). During the 1960s ECT was widely used as a treatment for severe depression. At Friern Hospital it was administered on 3 days every week. After receiving their sedative 'premed', the patients were lined up to await their treatment. When their turn came, they lay on a couch, an anaesthetic mask was held over their nose and mouth until they were unconscious, and electrodes were placed on their temples through which an electric shock was administered to induce an epileptic seizure. When the seizure was over and consciousness returned, the dazed patient was accompanied to a bed in the recovery area where he or she 'slept it off'. I thought then that it was the most barbaric treatment I had ever seen and my opinion on this has not changed over time. Despite my feelings, I have to admit that in many cases ECT was very effective, especially in patients for whom all other treatments had failed. Indeed, some patients who had received several courses of treatment spread across several months described it as a 'lifeline'.

The second ward, also kept locked, was a long-stay ward with 30 beds. This ward was equally shocking, although for different reasons. Most of the patients were labelled as 'burnt out schizophrenics' or were just old. Some had been inpatients for many years. One had been admitted 30 years before for no better reason than being rejected by her family after having an illegitimate child. One day I was approached at the ward door by a woman I thought was one of the patients from a 'better' ward. Patients from 'better' wards would be sent to other wards to do the washing up and the cleaning, in return for which they were given a small amount of pocket money that they could spend in the hospital shop. I opened the door for her and she took herself off to Brighton for the first day's 'freedom' she had known in years (her ability to do so with only her pocket money belied her so-called mental inadequacy) before turning up safe and sound at bed-time. I was severely disciplined, and I think if I had not been a mere 'student from the general' my nursing career might have come to an untimely end.

The long-stay ward was divided into two parts, one for daytime and one where the patients slept in a single row of beds barely 3 feet apart. Opposite the row of beds were two 'padded cells', which were now used as single rooms for sick patients, who were nursed on a mattress on the floor. If one could forget their original use, they were quite beautiful, with walls, ceiling and floor lined with the softest white kid. Most of the patients were incontinent at night – it would have been quite difficult for anyone to get out of bed and walk to the only toilet at the other end of the ward – and the stench of urine when one arrived on duty at 7am was overwhelming. Our first job each morning was to strip all the beds, get the patients into dry clothing provided by the hospital, so they 'fitted where they touched', and serve breakfast. Meals came to the ward in a heated trolley. Breakfast consisted of porridge, cereals, bread and margarine, and fried bacon and egg. The patients never got the bacon and egg, which was taken from the trolley and put to keep warm in the oven in the ward kitchen. After the patients had had their breakfast, the nurses repaired to the ward kitchen to enjoy this food. The rest of the day was spent giving out drugs, bathing patients in the ward's single bathroom according to the rota carefully worked out a month in advance in the ward's bathing book, getting patients ready for meals and clearing up afterwards, and just minding them to see that they did not harm themselves or anyone else. The only 'treatments' appeared to be enemas; activities or special events of any kind were rare.

An indication of the coming revolution in psychiatric care, however, was provided by my third placement at Friern. This was in the new unit called Halliwick, which was built outside the walls of the main hospital. Here, 30 patients of both sexes spent short periods of time during the acute phase of their illness in a therapeutic community staffed by doctors, nurses, social workers and therapists of various kinds. The consultant in charge of the unit was Dr Richard Hunter, who was committed to new ways of treating mentally ill patients. He opposed the use of ECT and psychosurgery, and pioneered gentler methods. The staff worked as a multidisciplinary team with the patients, talking through their problems in individual and group sessions, teaching them to build social relationships and helping them to re-learn the patterns of normal life that their illness had, sometimes quite drastically, interrupted. There were no locked doors, no keys and no uniforms. I was introduced to art and music therapy. Nursing here enabled me to develop an exciting new knowledge base and skills in listening, teaching and counselling, and the skills that I learnt at Friern Hospital have stayed with me always.

Living out and moving on

In our third year we were allowed to live out. A good deal of linen and food made the journey from UCH to the nurses' flats and back (well, the linen returned). I moved with a group of friends into a flat near to the tube station from where we could get to UCH in time to be on duty by 7.30am. There were seven of us and only six beds, one of which was a double, but since at least one of us would be on night duty and sleeping in the daytime while the others were at work, we managed. As the oldest, it fell to me to collect the rent from the others, to put out the rubbish and to try to keep the place clean. That was quite hard work, however, so when the lease ran out I decided to find a place of my own. I found an attic bed-sit near Kentish Town tube station, even nearer to UCH. Here the gas fire had to be fed with shillings but the electricity was included in the rent (2 guineas a week), so I spent time swotting for finals curled up in bed under an electric blanket.

Finals came and went. There were two sets of exams, one for the state-registered nurse (SRN) qualification, and then the hospital finals. I had no problem with examinations, and I managed to achieve the prize for highest marks in the hospital finals. The all-important letter pertaining to my SRN results was dated 26 November 1965:

Prize for the highest marks in the hospital final examination March 1966 (I still have, and use, the Pears Family Cookery!)

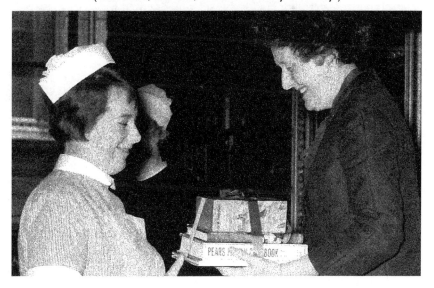

Dear Madam,
I have much pleasure in informing you that you have been successful in passing the Final State Examination for the General part of the Register held in October 1965. You are now eligible to apply for admission to this part of the Register on payment of a registration fee of £3 3s.0d.

Although the state finals were the ones that gave the SRN qualification, which was required to work as a qualified nurse, hospital finals were considered even more important, and completion of a further 'blue belt' year was required for the hospital badge and eligibility for membership of the Nurses' League. Once again I was in trouble. I had decided to go into health visiting, and had obtained a place to begin training starting in September 1966, but since my 'blue belt' year would not finish until October I would not be able to take up this place and would have to postpone it for a whole year. Moreover, I knew that before beginning health visitor training I would have to undertake some midwifery training, and since my only paediatric experience was the time I spent on ward 32 at the very beginning of my training, I felt I needed more experience with children.

Once again my RCN mentors came to my rescue. As part of my growing interest in health visiting and public health, I had met Renate Hiller, who was Director of Nursing of the London Borough of Camden. She offered me a job as a staff nurse in one of the borough day nurseries just behind Euston Station for 3 months until Christmas. I also obtained a place on the new shortened maternity nursing course, which started in January and met the entry requirement for health visitor training. The course was based in Reading, where Roger was already working and where we planned to live after we were married. It all came together nicely.

On being offered the job of staff nurse in Camden Borough and making my decision to leave UCH, I wrote my letter of resignation. I was duly summoned to Matron's office. It was a difficult interview, but perhaps Matron was glad to see the back of me. Her final words were: 'I hope, Miss Hickery, that one day you will be proud to say that you trained at UCH.' In response I dared reply, 'I hope, Matron, that perhaps one day you will be proud to say that I trained at UCH.' Some years later, when I was allowed to buy a hospital badge and was not only allowed to join the UCH Nurses' League but invited to be guest speaker at one of the League's annual meetings, I think we were reconciled. Perhaps, therefore, both of these hopes came true!

PART 2: THE DAY JOB

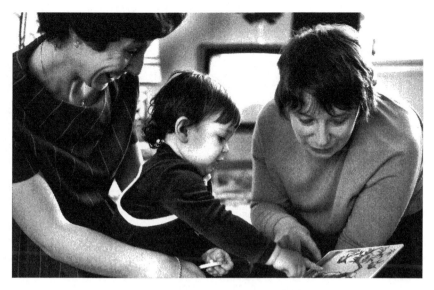

Health visiting in Berkshire 1967

CHAPTER 3: HAVING IT ALL

First career: Health visiting

In September 1966 I started my health visitor training at the Royal College of Nursing. Once again I was blessed to have excellent mentors in Claire Brookes and Norah Daniels, who were at this time among the leaders in the development of health visiting. The Council for the Education and Training of Health Visitors had been established as the new regulatory body for health visiting in 1962, and a curriculum intended to produce what became known as the 'new breed' health visitor had been introduced; I was one of the first of the new breed. The journal *Mother and Child* ran a special issue on the new training, to which I was invited to contribute an article with the title 'From a recent student's view'; it was the Editor of this journal who introduced me to Sylvia Hull, then Editor of *Mother and Baby*, a monthly news-stand magazine for which I continued to write for the next 10 years.

For my practical experience I was based at the Walmer Road Infant Welfare Centre in North Kensington. At that time North Kensington was a very deprived area consisting of long terraces and crescents of dilapidated, though once-magnificent, 19th century houses with peeling paintwork and 'fronts' full of dustbins, each house occupied by several families sharing inadequate kitchen and bathroom facilities located on the landings between floors. There was a high population of immigrants, mostly West Indian. Racial tensions were high: this was the scene of the Notting Hill riots and the year before Enoch Powell's 'Rivers of Blood' speech. At around 9am on weekdays a procession of tired-looking women in curlers could be seen pushing prams containing two or three children, with more children tagging along behind, headed towards the school. Later in the day the same women, still in curlers, would push those same prams laden with washing to and from the public washhouse in Silchester Road. Families of six or seven children were the norm. In addition to various observational visits, we students carried a caseload of eight families whom we visited throughout the year, and from whom we chose four as case studies to submit to the examiners. The written examination, which took place in June, was followed by 3 months' supervised practice in a different area, and then an oral examination in September. The training for health visiting was far more rigorous then than it has now become.

Our training included doing a project and writing a dissertation. My project concerned the role of the health visitor in family planning. In particular, it considered the question as to why families such as those in my caseload, who were desperately in need of family planning advice, did not get it and did not use the services that were available. The issue was topical and controversial because in 1967 the NHS (Family Planning) Act for the first time allowed local authorities to provide birth control advice regardless of marital status, on social as well as medical grounds. As part of my project I undertook training to become a qualified family planning nurse, and I became involved with the Family Planning Association's (FPA's) training programmes for health visitors and midwives (who were then employed by local authorities), and in the campaigning activities that eventually led to the inclusion of family planning services within the NHS in 1974. My project was published in the October 1967 issue of the FPA journal *Family Planning* – my first 'proper' publication.

I took up my post as a newly-qualified health visitor, employed by Berkshire County Council, in September 1967. I was attached to a group practice in Mortimer, a village a few miles south of Reading. The practice was a group of five GPs with about 11,000 patients in a mainly rural area covering two villages, Mortimer and Burghfield. The concepts of attachment to general practice and the primary health care team were just beginning. The practice had good purpose-built premises and was generally very forward looking. As an attached health visitor my caseload was the same as for all the others in the team: all of the patients registered with the practice. The range of work was wide. I visited families with babies and young children, older people, and followed up medico-social problems referred to me by the GPs and other members of the team. With the other health visitor member of the team I held baby clinics in the local church hall. I also monitored the local playgroups and childminders. With the midwife I ran antenatal and parenting classes, including a session for fathers. Under the new legislation the GPs obtained a grant from the local authority to provide a practice-based family planning clinic, which, as a qualified family planning nurse, I ran. I also started a course in personal relationships (otherwise known as sex education) with the final year boys and girls at the local comprehensive school, and published an account of it in *Nursing Times* under the title 'Learning for living'.

At that time, some of these activities were hugely innovative; for example, ours was probably the first practice-based family planning clinic. Similarly, sex education in secondary schools was rare. This was health visiting as I believe it should be. In 1973 some of our duties (e.g. responsibility for day care of children) were transferred to the new social services departments. Others, such as visiting older people, simply died away. I believe it is a tragedy that in the years since then the role and function of the health visitor has become increasingly limited, until it is in some places no more than a protocol-driven programme for mothers with babies.

The GPs were at first somewhat suspicious of the extended knowledge and broader range of skills possessed by this 'new breed' health visitor, especially a graduate! The most sceptical of them was won over when one day I visited a family with a 14-month-old baby who was just starting to walk, except that she ran rather than walked, and with an abnormal gait. When I examined her I could see that she probably had a unilateral congenital dislocation of one hip. The GPs prided themselves on knowing their patients – the obstetrician in the team had delivered many of them and watched them grow up to have their own babies. Somehow, however, this child's hip had been missed. At first the GP did not believe me, but I persuaded him to refer her for X-ray, and there it was. After that he always listened carefully to what I said. I soon became involved in the work of the Council for the Education and Training of Health Visitors as a member of the various working parties that were working on issues such as defining the role and function of the health visitor, development of the primary health care team, and attachment to general practice. I also worked closely with the RCN and the Royal College of General Practitioners, speaking at conferences and study days, publishing articles, and providing training on attachment and the primary health care team. In addition to this, I took part in several BBC television programmes on health visiting and the primary health care team.

In health visiting feedback does not come quickly, but it does come, sometimes in strange ways. Some months after I had left this job, I was standing in the checkout queue at our local Woolworths, when a voice behind me said: 'Goodness, I remember you; you saved my life!' I knew that that was not my kind of business, but when I turned round I recognised the woman and remembered her situation. Her baby, aged 8 months when I first met her, had just been diagnosed as having phenylketonuria, a rare genetic condition in which the baby cannot metabolise phenylalanine, and which, among other things, causes foul-smelling stools; if not diagnosed early enough (it should be detected at birth by a routine screening test) and treated, it causes brain damage and other problems. She and her husband were devastated; in particular her husband, a top scientist, could not face the prospect of a mentally handicapped child. When I visited her for the first time I found her in tears and up to her armpits in a sink of very smelly nappies (this was before the days of disposables) because the washing machine had broken down; the baby was refusing to eat the rather unpalatable special diet he had been prescribed; and her husband had retreated into his work. I had rolled up my sleeves and we talked as we washed the nappies together.

Sometimes, however, my enthusiasm and engagement backfired. One of my clients was a 17-year-old single mother who already had two children (by different fathers) and had just had her third. The two previous children had been in and out of hospital all their lives, usually with diarrhoea or respiratory infections. I was determined that this baby should reach its first birthday with no hospital admissions, so I visited frequently and focused intensively on the baby's nutrition and her bottle hygiene. A year later when I left to have my own first baby, her baby had had no hospital admissions. When I visited her for the last time she presented me with a beautiful bottle-feeding kit. It turned out that she had saved her benefits money for weeks to buy me this gift! I realised that I had gone too far in creating dependence, but at least the baby was healthy.

From October 1966, and for the first 5 years of our married life, we lived at Foxhill House, an all-male hall of residence on the Reading University campus (mixed halls were yet to come). Although we were only a few years older than the students, we were in loco parentis (a role that still operated in universities until the late 1960s) to 28 young men – and we loved it. We got to know them and their girlfriends and enjoyed being part of the group. I became the unpaid health visitor to the whole community. I remember one evening coming home late after an antenatal class at the surgery to find half a dozen students sharing a beer with Roger, and showing them the film of the birth of a baby – to which one agriculture student responded drily: 'Well it's much less complicated with cows!' Whether it was 'Can you spare some sugar because my girlfriend is making a cake?' or 'June, my girlfriend's pregnant', I was doing health visiting all through that time. The orientation and skills that I used during those early years as a health visitor have stayed with me all through my career

Second career: Author and journalist

When Andrew was born in February 1969, and then Gillian in January 1972, my personal and professional lives became totally intertwined. Without a 'regular' job, I at least had flexibility.

Andrew did not interfere with my other activities – since he had to follow his food supply I took him everywhere with me. Even when Gillian was born 3 years later, thanks to the support of a wonderful husband and a network of good neighbours I was able continue my involvement with the Royal College of Nursing, to finish my MPhil, and continue writing and publishing. For example, as a health visitor I had been running antenatal classes for other people, so now I decided to test what I had taught there against my own experience. When I was pregnant with Andrew, I decided to attend both the classes at the hospital where I was booked for delivery and the classes in psycho-prophylaxis run by the National Childbirth Trust, which at that time was becoming popular. I compared them and wrote about them in the *Nursing Mirror*; and I wrote about my experience of labour – which was long, hard, but fortunately normal – in another *Nursing Mirror* article called 'It's different on the receiving end'.

It certainly was different on the receiving end. My mother had died the previous year and Roger's mother was 100 miles away, so we were on our own. When Andrew was about a week old, Roger came home from work to find me in tears. 'Why can't I stop him crying,' I sobbed, 'I'm a health visitor, I'm supposed to be able to!' The lesson, which was repeated many times later, is that when health professionals become patients they are just as vulnerable as anyone else. I remember how horrified I was when, much later, I was worried about Gillian, and I saw her medical notes with 'Mother is SRN, do not visit' blazoned in large letters across the cover.

At about this time, Sylvia Hull, Editor of *Mother and Baby*, was looking for someone to write an article about health visitors for her general readership and was given my name. I wrote the article, then another, and then another. Within a very short time I was writing a regular monthly article as the magazine's Health Visitor Consultant. A few months later I added the role of Agony Aunt, answering readers' letters at £1 per letter. The role expanded further, and soon I was writing factsheets and leaflets for readers with titles such as Tinies on the Move, Successful Breastfeeding, Feeding Toddlers, and Potty Training. I translated the packet instructions for Milupa baby foods when they were first introduced into the UK from Switzerland. I wrote a booklet on premenstrual tension, which was used as evidence in a court case in support of a woman charged with shoplifting, and a book called *Family Health and Safety* as one of a series produced by the Co-op available to customers for 65p plus two labels from any Co-op products! I also wrote the leaflets that accompanied the monthly toy offerings of the Early Learning Centre when it was just a one-man band mail-order company. How I wished I had bought shares when it became a big company! I think I did more and better health visiting through *Mother and Baby* than ever I did in a normal health visitor job.

These efforts helped us to pay the mortgage, but there were other benefits too. Manufacturers of baby products would send us samples to try out and keep, hoping for a favourable review: I tested the first Maclaren baby buggy, the early disposable nappies, new baby foods, and various bits of baby equipment. We had a free trip to Menorca, where I advised a hotel how to set up a crèche for guests' children, and a trip to Legoland in Denmark where we visited the factory to see how Lego was made. The biggest benefit of all, however, was the constant (constructive) criticism of my monthly articles by Sylvia Hull. I would send her my monthly article, which she would send back covered in red ink, and the cycle would be repeated several times until she was satisfied. She taught me most of what I know about the craft of writing – a skill that has stood me in good stead ever since.

I continued to write for professional journals, and I published several books. I wrote several editorials for the *Health and Social Services Journal* and the nursing section of their regular feature 'Leading Opinion', usually arguing the nursing perspective on some controversial issue. In the *Nursing Times* of 2 July 1970, I responded to a letter from a doctor who was attacking nursing's aspirations arising out of the Salmon Report. I wrote:

Madam,
I am the very model of a modern Surgeon General,
I've knowledge and experience both surgical and medical,
I'm an expert with the scalpel and in modern physiology,
I know about the newest drugs and Freudian psychology.
I'm very well acquainted too with nurses' ways professional,
I've heard of Mr Salmon and I've read of Florence Nightingale,
In short, in things professional both surgical and medical,
I am the very model of a modern surgeon general.
In fact, when I have learnt that nurses aren't my handmaids personal,
But colleagues, and of nurses too, just like their partners medical,
There's some excel in bedside skills, and some administration,
Like doctors, some elect to train to manage their own station.
For lay administration shouldn't rule a true profession;
I forget that this applies for nursing too – that's my confession.
In short, when I stick to medicine, abjure my doctor's arrogance,
You'll find no better surgeon, nurse, attendance than on whom to dance.
For my expertise in nursing, though I know I'm quite a clever guy,
Has only been brought down to the beginning of the century.
But in expertise professional, both surgical and medical,
I am the very model of a modern surgeon general.
Nurses:
'Tis sad that in deciding nursing policy professional,
He is the very model of a modern surgeon general.
With apologies to W.S. Gilbert but none to J.K. McCollum

Later, *The Times* newspaper, having established the *Times Educational Supplement* and the *Times Literary Supplement*, decided to launch a *Times Health Supplement*. The Editor was Jill Turner, who, when *The Times* decided that it was no longer commercially viable, re-launched it as a monthly briefing. For 6 years in every issue I wrote a column called 'Nursing Matters' until it finally died in 1987.

Mother and Baby gave me a wonderful account of the next few years. It so happened that Deputy Editor Máire Messenger was due to have her second child at about the same time as Gillian was due to be born, so every month for 3 years the magazine ran a column called 'Diary of Two Babies'. One month Máire would write about Hannah's progress and I would comment by writing about Gillian; and the next month I would write first about Gillian and Máire would follow up with her account about Hannah. The purpose was to show how all children follow the same developmental stages but at different speeds and in different ways, and to offer practical tips derived from our accounts of how we were coping. We developed a following akin, in the days before Facebook, to Mumsnet. Lots of readers joined in with accounts of their children's progress.

Most of my accounts were happy, but the 'Diary' records some poignant moments too. When Gillian was just 8 months old she was admitted to hospital with pneumonia, which developed into meningitis. For the ninth month 'Diary', I wrote: 'Gillian is in hospital. I am writing this month's Diary at her bedside. At the moment she is sleeping peacefully, pink and rosy although her breathing is still very fast. She has broncho-pneumonia.' For the 10th month 'Diary' I wrote:

This has been a terrible month for us all. Gillian is still in hospital. She came home on Tuesday, rather pale and wan, and a good deal more subdued than before her illness, but with her chest clear, her temperature normal, and her infection apparently cured. She continued to have antibiotic medicine, and was a little stronger each day until Saturday. On Saturday morning she was again very lethargic, very reluctant to eat or drink, or even to be touched; she seemed to want only to be left alone to sleep. The doctor came and could find nothing specific to account for her lethargy. He came again on Sunday. On Monday, since she was no better, I asked if she could be re-admitted to hospital. The doctor who examined her on admission could find nothing specific. I began to think there was something wrong with me. The doctor was very sympathetic about my 'neurotic mother syndrome' and agreed to keep Gillian for 24 hours 'for observation'. Although I had stayed in the hospital with her the first time, this time I went home, feeling that this would permit a better assessment of her condition. By the time I arrived at the hospital the next day, she was obviously very much worse, and tests which had been carried out during the morning showed that she now had meningitis.... Once again I moved into the little cubicle. All that night I was terrified that she was going to die. I asked about having her christened, and felt guilty that we just hadn't got round to it before. The night nurses plied me with coffee and moral support until by about 3am I was able to sleep. I woke again at 6am when the nurse came to give Gillian an injection and take her temperature. Gillian was crying but the sound was the most wonderful music I ever heard, because it was her normal lusty bellow and not the high pitched squeal which is typical of meningitis and which she had been making the previous day.

I have reflected on this episode many times, and tried to draw out the lessons I learned, both for myself and for other mothers. I had a huge post-bag of letters from *Mother and Baby* readers, often sharing similar experiences, and some expressing for the first time, they said, feelings that they had never expressed before. Some feelings I did not write in the 'Diary'. I shall never forget telling myself as I drove to the hospital that I was just a 'neurotic mother' – how many times have I heard other mothers described that way? – and then my horror when I saw Gillian in her cot, obviously very ill. The nurse said, 'Oh Mrs Clark, we've done some tests and the doctor will want to see you.' I turned to ice. I just picked Gillian up and held her to me, and thought of every fatal illness I knew about. When the doctor said it was meningitis I was almost relieved. At least that was something I could get my head around. Later I worked nights as a bank nurse on that ward, and was able to share a little of what other mothers were feeling. Health-care practitioners must always, always listen to what a mother says – if she says something is wrong, it usually is.

The 34th month records how Andrew was knocked down by a car outside his school. Both bones in his lower left leg were broken, but thankfully there were no other injuries. The fractures were set under a general anaesthetic and Andrew was admitted to the same ward as Gillian had been in almost 3 years earlier. Once again I moved in too. At 3am he woke and wanted to talk about the accident. I was so glad I was there to listen. I was able to write about the importance of facilities for mothers to be admitted with their children, about the guilt that mothers experience when their children have an accident, and about the effect that such episodes can have on other siblings. Once again my post-bag was huge.

Third career: Nursing research

When in the summer of 1968 I became pregnant with Andrew, I had to give up my job because in those days it was expected and there were few part-time job opportunities and few childcare facilities, but I did not give up working. In July of that year the 'Report of the Committee on Local Authority and Allied Personal Social Services' (the Seebohm Report) was published. It proposed that the various local government welfare services of the time be brought together into integrated social services departments with a central role for social workers. In doing so it removed from health visitors functions they regarded as theirs, such as the registration and supervision of nurseries, playgroups and childminders. Social workers were delighted but health visitors were furious. They complained that their role and function were undervalued and misunderstood. I agreed, and stood up on several conference platforms to say so; but I did argue that if people did not understand what health visitors did, it was probably because health visitors had not told them. There was a plethora of reports, recommendations and articles in professional journals about what the role of the health visitor should be, but a dearth of factual information about the actual content and practice of health visiting. I argued that what was needed was some proper research.

I was one of very few health visitors with a degree, which was a university requirement for undertaking postgraduate research. I was also currently (being pregnant) unemployed, and living in a university. I obtained a grant from the (then) King Edward's Hospital Fund for London – the first one given to an individual nurse – and started to do what became my MPhil thesis. The result was a study of health visiting in Berkshire. My sample was the population of health visitors employed by Berkshire County Council – 82 in all. I sent a questionnaire to every health visitor and got a response rate of 89.1%. I interviewed 79 health visitors and persuaded 72 to record all their home visits for a week using a recording form that I devised. These amounted to 2057 visits in all.

I knew nothing about research methods, but I had tremendous goodwill: I discovered that being accompanied by a breast-fed baby (Andrew was born at the beginning of the fieldwork period) established an immediate rapport with health visitor interviewees. There was no-one qualified to take on my

M.Phil graduation, Reading University, July 1972

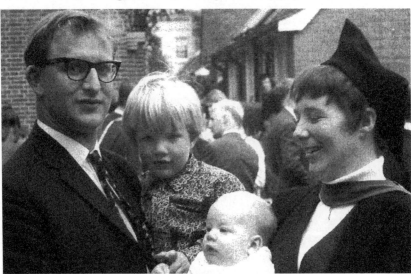

supervision because there were almost no nurses with postgraduate degrees, but Professor of Politics Peter Campbell and Dr Viola Klein, Reader in the Department of Sociology, agreed to be my formal supervisors, with the warning that since they knew nothing about the field I would have to get my 'content' supervision wherever I could find it. I drew on my network of mentors including Marjory Simpson, Jean McFarlane and Grace Owen, and the fledgling RCN Research Discussion Group. Professor Margot Jefferys, one of the founders of the developing field of medical sociology, became my external examiner. I graduated in July 1972, saying it had taken two babies for me to complete the work! (Gillian having been born in January 1972.) The thesis was published in book form in 1973 under the title *A Family Visitor*, the first in the series of research monographs published through the 1970s by the RCN in conjunction with the DHSS. It seemed to make a great impact; I did not know whether to be pleased or horrified when I found that it was still included in the reading lists for student health visitors 30 years later! It was also published as an article in 1976 in the very first issue of the *Journal of Advanced Nursing*.

Although I had now completed my MPhil degree, I recognised that I still knew almost nothing about research methods, and I had searched in vain for some kind of course that would be compatible with my family responsibilities. Then I heard that Surrey University was starting a part-time course leading to an MSc in social research that was specially geared for social workers and NHS staff. Guildford was only an hour's train journey away from home, and attendance was required on only 1 day a week, so I enrolled. The course was run by the Department of Sociology, and in addition to social research methods we were introduced to the disciplines of social policy and medical sociology. When the *Journal of Advanced Nursing* was launched in 1976, I submitted an essay I had written as an assignment on the sociology of organisations; based on the work of the sociologist Robert Michels, who showed how in political parties the full-time officials were always more powerful than the part-time elected leaders, it was called 'Functions and dysfunctions in a professional association: The case of the Royal College of Nursing'. It was strangely prophetic.

It is difficult now to remember how technology has developed. We were asked to provide some of our own textbooks and equipment, the most expensive item of which (costing a lot of money) was a calculator. As part of the statistics course we learned how to analyse data using the new university computer, which was so huge that it occupied a whole building on campus.

At the end of the first year we had written examinations and chose the topic for our dissertations. I was still deeply involved in the debates about childbirth and the work of the National Childbirth Trust and still writing for *Mother and*

Baby, so I decided to look at mothers' and midwives' experiences of childbirth, testing the hypothesis that the better the mother–midwife communication, the better the mother's experience. From my early observations, however, a quite different picture emerged. I found that both mothers and midwives could be categorised as 'high tech' or 'low tech': when a low tech midwife delivered a low tech mother (i.e. one who wanted a natural birth with minimal intervention) the mother's satisfaction was high; when a high tech midwife (i.e. one who favoured intervention such as epidural) delivered a low tech mother, the mother was very dissatisfied; when a low tech midwife delivered a high tech mother (who wanted maximum intervention) the mother was very dissatisfied; but when a high tech midwife or a doctor delivered a high tech mother, the mother was very satisfied, even when things went wrong and the delivery was very traumatic. In other words, the key factor was not the quality of communication but the mother's expectations and wishes.

I never got the chance to complete the study because soon after I started I was approached by the Department of Health to do more work on health visiting. In spite of my earlier work and the work of others, the Department of Health still claimed not to know what health visitors did. I therefore started a new study, which eventually became my PhD. Supported by a DHSS grant, I took up an appointment as Research Fellow at what was then the Polytechnic of the South Bank, now South Bank University. The Head of Department was Grace Owen, herself a leader in health visiting education and politics, and she headed a department with a strong track record of health visitor training and development. Grace was a visionary and pioneer in nursing education whose contribution was never fully appreciated. She was one of the small band of nurse educators, which included Jean McFarlane and Christine Chapman, who pioneered degree programmes in nursing during the 1960s. The Association of Integrated and Degree Courses in Nursing, which brought this group of nurse leaders together, was eventually subsumed within the RCN and, sadly, much of its work now appears to have been lost.

I appointed as my research assistant Kate Robinson, then a newly-qualified health visitor who later became a professor and dean at the University of Luton, and then Deputy Vice Chancellor of the University of Bedfordshire. Kate perhaps more than anyone else epitomises the challenges of 'having it all' – during her time as my research assistant she had three babies!

The research that eventually became my (and Kate's) PhD broke new ground in a number of ways. The Department of Health and health visitors themselves were still complaining that health visiting was not understood. The health visitors argued that this was because such data as were available came from surveys undertaken by people who were not health visitors and therefore asked the wrong questions and misinterpreted the replies. The Department of Health saw the solution as a qualitative study undertaken by a health visitor, i.e. me, the purpose of which was to develop a more valid survey instrument. I set up a study in which health visitors tape-recorded their home visits, the tapes were transcribed, and the information divided into categories that would be developed so they could be used more widely in 'better' surveys.

The use of tape recorders in research is now commonplace, but in those days was rare; it had never been done in health visiting. It was especially problematic because health visiting conversations are conducted in the client's own home, so the ethical issues around confidentiality and privacy were considerable. There were also methodological questions about whether dyadic interaction, i.e. between the client and the health visitor, would be changed by the presence of a third person (triadic interaction) if one were used to manage the machine. In pilot studies we tested the alternative methods, and eventually decided that the health visitors would manage the machines themselves, having already obtained the client's consent, turning the machine on before they entered the home and off after they left. The health visitors were also asked to briefly explain the purpose of the visit before they entered and to reflect on it after they left. The health visitors recorded their visits to selected families over the period of 1 year from the birth of a new baby. This method resulted in several problems of data quality – sometimes the machine did not work, or the battery ran out, or the sound was muffled by extraneous noise. The good news, however, was that we generated enough data from enough health visitors to transcribe and analyse. The very good news was that for the first time ever we had some 'specimens' of health visiting that we could examine again and again in the same way that other scientists might examine a specimen in a test tube.

Transcription took ages, but the real problem began with the analysis. We divided each transcript into 'episodes' and began to categorise the episodes according to the topic being discussed. We assumed, wrongly, that having identified the topic it would be easy to develop a coding system and to code each topic ready for computerised analysis. But we were unable to achieve inter-coder reliability. By the beginning of 1981 I was ready to give up. The Department of Health money had run out, and most important of all I desperately wanted to get back to health visiting practice.

One of the benefits of working in an academic environment had been that I had time to read about new developments in nursing and had the opportunity to discuss them with academic colleagues. In particular, one of the new ideas crossing the Atlantic was the use of the nursing process.

Health visitors at this time were still arguing that health visiting was not nursing but was a distinct profession in its own right, and therefore this new-fangled approach to nursing had nothing to offer them. I have always seen health visiting as part of nursing, and I was very attracted to this logical and structured approach to practice. I wanted to try it out to see if it could work in health visiting so I applied for and obtained a part-time health visiting post back home in Reading, to start in September 1981.

Before September, however, there were things to do. Even though in my view my PhD project had failed, I recognised the importance of the unique methodological approach we had developed, so I wrote about this in the *Health Visitor* journal. A few weeks later I received a letter from Jean McFarlane in Manchester: 'I saw your article in the *Health Visitor* journal. Interesting. Now what about this PhD?' To this I replied: 'I've given it up. You win some and you lose some. But I'm back in practice now and I've got a far more interesting problem that I would like to come and discuss with you.' The problem was that in the absence of forms or 'headings' of the kind that are now common in structured nursing documentation, I could not find an assessment framework that would work for health visiting. I tried the system that doctors used, based on body systems; I tried the frameworks offered by the new 'grand theory models' such as Roper, Tierney and Logan and those that were also crossing the Atlantic at this time. Nothing worked. They all focused on the patient as an individual whereas the health visiting 'client' is a family group; and they all presupposed a 'problem' needing treatment, whereas health visiting is much more about maintaining 'normality'.

I went to Manchester and poured it all out to Jean. After listening patiently for several hours she said: 'You idiot! The reason you can't get inter-coder reliability in your research is the same as the reason why you can't find an assessment framework in your practice. Everybody intuitively and subconsciously sorts data according to a mental model or paradigm that they have in their head, although it is rarely made explicit. Your coders are all using different models which are not made explicit; and in looking for a framework for assessment you are struggling to find a model for health visiting which similarly has never been made explicit. Your task is to develop a model which can describe and explain health visiting practice. Moreover, you have in your transcripts the raw material you need to do it. You need to re-analyse your data in a completely different way, perhaps using the new ideas [which were also at that time crossing the Atlantic] about how to build a model – first identify the key concepts, explore them, put them together showing the relationships between them, and then test it out in practice.'

So that is what I did, and that is what became – albeit 4 years later (in 1985) – my PhD. The model worked. It was published as 'A model for health visiting' in Kershaw and Salvage's 1986 book *Models for Nursing*. I regret now that I did not publish it more widely, but before I could do so I took up, and became totally immersed in, my new post at Guy's and Lewisham.

From health visiting to primary health care

The year 1981 was significant for me in several ways. First, there was the decision to return to practice. Then, in the gap between leaving South Bank and starting back in health visiting practice, two events completely changed my outlook on health visiting and primary health care. Both derived from the World Health Organization (WHO) Declaration of Alma Ata of 1978, which set the goal of 'Health for All by the Year 2000', and identified the redirection of health services to focus on primary health care as the means of achieving it. I totally took on board the WHO concept of primary health care as: 'essential health care; based on practical, scientifically sound, and socially acceptable method and technology; universally accessible to all in the community through their full participation; at an affordable cost; and geared toward self-reliance and self-determination.'

Over the next few years I worked with the International Council of Nurses (ICN) in a programme of workshops for nurses from across Europe on 'Nursing in Support of Health for All', and in the RCN we initiated a position statement on nursing in primary health care that set out the WHO definition, nursing's contribution, and what the RCN was doing. The watchword was Dr Halfden Mahler's call: 'If the millions of nurses in a thousand different places articulate the same ideas and convictions about PHC [primary health care] and come together as one force then they could act as a powerhouse for change.' Later I used 'Powerhouse for Change' as the title for the work I did to bring all the community nursing specialist groups within the RCN together as the Community Nursing Association.

Some 20 years later, when I was teaching a class of nursing undergraduates about primary health care, I asked the class why the UK had never adopted the WHO strategy, in particular its underlying philosophy, but had instead gone down the road of 'primary care' of which the business model was the independent contractor status of the GP and where the central character was the GP. The answer I was looking for was that in 1979 Mrs Thatcher became Prime Minister and her new right-wing ideology precluded notions such as solidarity and collectivism. There was silence for a while, and then a hand in the back row went up and a voice said: 'Well that was the year that I was born!'

Primary health care in Scandinavia

The first event that changed my outlook was being awarded a Council of Europe Fellowship to look at primary health care and community nursing services in Scandinavia. I visited Finland and Denmark. Once again my RCN networks, this time Dame Sheila Quinn and Jean McFarlane, opened doors that I would otherwise have not even known about. Dame Sheila arranged for me to spend some time with her friend Ingrid Hamelin, who was at that time Chief Nurse for the city of Helsinki. She arranged for me to 'shadow' health visitors in Helsinki and to talk with the country's influential leaders in primary health care. I spent a week with a health visitor in Varkaus, shadowing her work. I spent time with Professor Sirkka Lauri, a public health nurse and one of the country's first professors of nursing. Sirkka had studied under Jean at Manchester, and as almost the only two public health nurses in Europe who were working at doctoral level we became good friends, sent our children to stay with each other's families for holidays, and remained in close touch for many years.

What I saw in Finland bowled me over. The healthcare system was solidly based on primary health care, in which the public health nurses were seen and respected as the key leaders. Their practice was recognisable as having the same goals as health visiting in the UK, but they worked very differently. Every village had a well-equipped purpose-built health centre, which the nurse used as her base, and for their home visits the nurses carried portable weighing scales so their examinations of babies and children were much more rigorous than ours. I was still running baby clinics in church halls, which were too cold to allow babies to be undressed. Home visits were by appointment, while UK health visitors still visited randomly as if to 'catch out' families. I was particularly impressed by their documentation systems, which were shared with clients. These documents included percentile charts years before they became available in the UK and parent-held 'baby books'; this greatly influenced my own later work on nursing documentation. Along the way I tried saunas, followed by rolling in the snow, cross-country skiing, and joining in the Vappu celebrations on 1 May. The stereotype of Finnish people as 'cold' is quite untrue; I have visited Finland several times since 1981, and I think Finland is perhaps my favourite European country, after Wales of course.

The ICN Congress

The second view-changing event was that I attended the ICN Quadrennial Congress, held that year in Los Angeles, which was on the theme of 'Health for All: Challenge for Nursing'. It was my first visit to the USA, and I hated Los Angeles so much that I vowed never to go back.

Two things in particular stand out in my memory. The first was being accompanied to my room on arrival by a porter who said, 'Are you one of the nurses? Will you look at this lump in my mouth and tell me if it's bad. I can't afford to go to the doctor.' The second was sitting in the main hall along with 3000 other nurses awaiting the start of the opening session. To the nurse sitting next to me I said: 'Hello, I'm June, and I'm from the UK.' She replied: 'Hi! I'm Lyn. I'm local. I'm a nurse practitioner in primary health care.' I was astounded when she told me about her work. It was very like my work as a health visitor. Like most health visitors of the time I had been brought up to believe that health visiting was unique to the UK; I now know that almost every country has some kind of health visitor, usually called a public health nurse, and that we can learn a great deal from these colleagues in other countries. I stayed in touch with Lyn for several years, and learning more about her work contributed greatly to our work a few years later on developing the nurse practitioner role in the UK.

Back in the UK

Back in the UK I tried to share something of what I had learnt, but with limited success. In an article for the *Nursing Mirror* I commented that in the years I had been away from practice health visiting had become much more defensive and protectionist than it used to be. I challenged the way that health visitors tried to disassociate themselves from nursing, the practice of visiting families without warning, and the tradition that records should never be taken out of the office into a home or seen by a client. Health visitors were horrified at the idea of visiting by appointment, as I had seen in Finland. A health-visiting manager wrote to the *Nursing Mirror* saying that she would doubt the standards of practice of a health visitor who worked in this way.

Research career continued

Meanwhile I continued my research career. In 1982 I was asked to develop and deliver a research methods course for nurses in Durban, South Africa. Apartheid was still in operation, and the problem was that whereas white nurses could go to the UK or USA for advanced nursing education, black nurses could not; the solution was to take it to them. A 1-month course was arranged at the University of Durban, where the Department of Nursing, headed by Noelle Hunt and Heidi Brookes – both well-known anti-apartheid activists – was seen as an oasis of racial integration. I felt I could not do it alone, but most of the people whom I approached as partners refused because of apartheid. Finally Caroline Cox (later Baroness Cox

61

of Queensbury), then Director of the Nursing Education Research Unit at Chelsea College of the University of London, agreed to partner me. Apart from the success of the course itself, the highlight for me was seeing how community nurses delivered primary health care in rural areas outside the city. A small team consisting of a public health nurse, a nursing assistant, and a driver/technician would take a little white van equipped with a fridge and a small generator out into the bush. I remember in particular the health education competition where community nursing teams used songs, drama, and role-play to get across messages about topics such as breast feeding, family nutrition and home safety, and the open-air 'clinic' under a tree where the whole community brought their babies to be immunised.

Continuing my PhD

I continued with my PhD research under the supervision of Jean McFarlane and Grace Owen. I spoke at conferences and published several articles about the 'framework' I was developing. However, it was not until I was invited to participate in a WHO meeting on children and family breakdown held in Kiel in 1984 that I 'found' the theoretical framework that held all the pieces together. What I found was Antonovsky's 'salutogenic' model, which asked the question not what makes us sick but what, in the same adverse circumstances, keeps us healthy, and uses systems theory and the concept of 'generalised resistance resources' to provide an answer. The mechanism for maintaining the dynamic equilibrium called 'health' in the presence of internal and external stressors was 'coping', which was the most common key concept used by my research health visitors to explain and evaluate their visits to families. I tested the model in my own practice and it worked. I completed my thesis and graduated in 1985. I was proud to be the South Bank's first PhD in nursing.

Meanwhile I continued to work part time as a health visitor in Reading. This time I was attached to a not-very-good two-man general practice. There was none of the teamwork that had been so important in my previous practice. The doctors did not provide any 'out of hours service' so I gave 'my' families my telephone number. This was frowned upon by my managers, but my families never abused it.

I continued to pursue my interest in the nursing process, and I developed a way of documenting my practice, which I published under the title 'A way to get organised' based on the problem-oriented medical record or POMR and the subjective, objective, assessment, plan (SOAP) framework originally developed by Lawrence Weed. I adapted SOAP to become SOAPIER (Said,

Observed, Assessment, Plan, Intervention, Evaluation, Revision). I did not realise then the significance of this idea for my later work on nursing documentation and the study of nursing outcomes.

In 1983 the District Nursing Officer for West Berkshire, Roy Cubbin, whom I had got to know well, asked if I could help with the development of research awareness among the District's nurses. Following the publication of the Briggs Report the importance of research in nursing was increasingly being recognised, and I had recently been involved in the development of the RCN's new Daphne Heald Research Unit. Would I accept a post as Senior Nurse (Research) based in the School of Nursing? I said that I would, provided that I could continue with my health visiting practice. The School of Nursing staff members were not thrilled by what they saw as the imposition of an outsider, and my teaching about research, which I believed should have been at the very beginning of the pre-registration programme and integrated into all subjects, was limited to a single lecture in the study days the newly-qualified nurses had while waiting for their finals results.

It was not easy to work in two different management structures, or to divide the days of the week neatly between two jobs. However, opportunity was provided by pressure to develop standards for nursing practice. I had been a member of the RCN's Working Party on Standards of Care, chaired by Sheila Quinn, which had used the format developed by the American Nurses Association and had published two documents, *Standards of Nursing Care* and *Towards Standards*, in 1980 and 1981 respectively. The RCN work had fallen into abeyance when the responsible staff member, David Rye, left for another post and there was a gap before his successor was appointed. I was able to take what I had learnt in the RCN and use it to develop a similar system for Berkshire. Helen Kendall, who had been the District's Nursing Process Co-ordinator (a post created in all districts as the result of the decision by the General Nursing Council a few years earlier requiring the nursing process to be incorporated into the pre-registration curriculum and used as the organising framework for nursing practice), worked with me on this. Helen was a superb facilitator and teacher, and she continued the work on standards when I left Berkshire in 1985 for a post in London.

Having it all

Other than my first post in health visiting, my 50 years in nursing has been not a single career, but has comprised at least five: the first in health visiting, the second as an author and journalist, the third in nursing research, the fourth in nursing management, and the fifth in nursing education. Woven through all of these like the warp and weft of a rich tapestry has been my involvement in health politics and the RCN and my role as a wife and mother of two children. My career was never planned – it was just that as opportunities arose they seemed to be too good to miss! Paradoxically, the limitations of motherhood and family responsibilities also provided opportunities that I would not otherwise have had. The key was that I had much greater flexibility than a 'proper' (i.e. full-time) job would have permitted. I could continue my research and I could publish. I could attend meetings, and this, combined with my RCN connections, enabled me to serve as a member of several important policy committees. For example, for me the 1974 reorganisation of the NHS provided a wonderful opportunity. The new management arrangements, which were set out in great detail in a manual known as the Grey Book, included the provision that the newly-created Area Health Authorities must include a nurse member. Thanks no doubt to my RCN connections, I was appointed the nurse member of Berkshire Area Health Authority, on which I served for 10 years, and then to the Oxfordshire District Health Authority for a further 2. For the next 12 years I was deeply involved in the NHS in the role now labelled non-executive director. In Berkshire I worked closely with the Area Health Authority Executive Team and the two District Management Teams, especially with the directors of nursing (then called district nursing officers), and I represented the Area Health Authority on the Local Authority Social Services Committee, among others. In Oxfordshire I was involved with the exciting developments in nursing that were taking place there. If I had been employed in the NHS at this time it would have been at the very junior level of a staff nurse or field-level health visitor, whereas I had the opportunity to observe and participate in life at the top; I learned a great deal.

In Berkshire, one local initiative for which I was responsible was the establishment of one of the first nurse banks. Such arrangements are now common, but in those days had not generally been thought of. The bank enabled me to work Saturday nights as a staff nurse, while Roger was able to look after the children the next day while I slept. One day during lunch with the children, who were about 6 and 3 at the time, the conversation turned to what they wanted to be when they grew up. Andrew's aspirations were quite clear – he was going to be a footballer. Gillian thought for a minute, then said, 'I think I would like to be a nurse.' Somewhat bemused, I asked why. 'Because,' she said, 'nurses only have to work one night a week.'

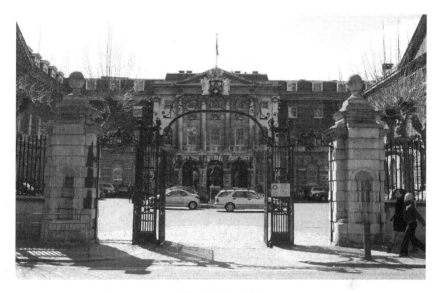

Guy's Hospital

CHAPTER 4: ROOM AT THE TOP?

In 1979 Mrs Thatcher became Prime Minister and the whole world changed. Everything was turned upside down. Over the next decade the application of the 'new right' ideology was gradually extended throughout the public sector, including the NHS and higher education, both of which led to fundamental changes in nursing. The most significant changes for nursing were the Griffiths Report of 1983, which led to the introduction of general management in the NHS, and specifically into nursing, and the NHS and Community Care Act 1990. The Act introduced the internal market into the NHS by means of the 'purchaser–provider split' between health authorities (the purchasers) and the newly-established NHS trusts (the providers). It was also brought into nursing education by the use of contracts between employers (the new NHS trusts) and education providers (i.e. the universities). For my own personal career, the changes in community care, and in particular the Cumberlege Report on community nursing, were also significant.

Guy's and Lewisham 1985–6

By 1984 I knew that it was time to move on from Berkshire, but I was not sure where or what to move to. The children were now old enough for me to consider a 'career' post but I was getting conflicting advice. One of my mentors was Malcolm Ross, then District Nursing Officer in Oxfordshire, under whose leadership great developments in nursing were taking shape in the form of a totally new approach to nursing in the establishment of a Nursing Development Unit at Burford. He advised avoiding a management post in favour of an expert advisory post, if I could find one. Most others said that I would have to go through the hoops of at least a 'number 7' management post first, even if I hated the thought of spending my days on such things as approving expenses forms. I applied for one of the (rare) advisory posts in a neighbouring area health authority, but it went to an internal candidate for whom it had obviously been specially created. Two re-organisations of the community nursing management structures in Berkshire provided several number 7 posts for which I applied – without success. I began to look further afield, and I applied for one in Hounslow and Spelthorne, which I thought was just within commuting range of Reading. Once again I was shortlisted and interviewed, but at the end of the day the nurse manager telephoned me to say that I had not been appointed, adding: 'It seems such a pity, June, because you've obviously got a lot to offer, but we didn't think you would "fit" in Hounslow and Spelthorne.' I was already quite sure that I would not 'fit' into Hounslow and Spelthorne, and probably not into any other traditional hierarchical structure.

About a week later over lunch at an RCN Council meeting I was regaling a few friends with this story, not noticing a woman eating her lunch at the other end of the table. I knew the woman only slightly as the representative of the Nursing Management Association on Council. Jo Plant was Chief Nursing Officer of Guy's and Lewisham Health Authority. She leaned across the table and said: 'I think I could do with someone like you. Come and see me.' I was about to leave the next day for the ICN Congress in Israel, but we made a date for my return a fortnight hence. When I arrived home from Israel, there was a package of information about Guy's and Lewisham, including its innovative plans for redeveloping community-based services supported by a new Griffiths'-style management structure. I thought this would be interesting to discuss so I went to see her, and within a week I received a letter offering me a 1-year post as Special Projects Officer. Guy's and Lewisham was at this time seen as the flagship for the new reforms. Guy's Hospital had merged with Lewisham Hospital and its accompanying psychiatric and community services to become a 'first-wave' NHS trust. The management structure was being re-organised to create a priority care unit, which covered psychiatric services, traditional community nursing services, mental handicap services (as they were then called), and services for older people. The challenge for psychiatric and mental handicap services was to close down the large 'bins' that currently provided long-term care for psychiatric and mentally handicapped patients and, in accordance with the new philosophy and arrangements for community-based care, to replace them with a number of community-based group homes. For services for older people, one of the projects – my job – was to develop a NHS nursing home. The concept of the NHS nursing home was introduced by the Royal Commission on the NHS (Merrison Report) published in 1979 and followed up in the Department of Health report *Growing Older* published in 1981. The commissioners, who included Jean McFarlane, had been impressed by what they saw in ways of caring for older people when they visited Denmark. Following the *Growing Older* report, three experimental NHS nursing homes were established in Plymouth, Blackpool and Sheffield. We visited the Plymouth home several times and modelled our new home on what we learned from the staff there. St Olave's Nursing Home was created by the conversion of the outpatients' department of St Olave's Hospital in Bermondsey, an old workhouse hospital that had just been closed. It was not an ideal building, but we tried to establish the values, attitudes, and physical facilities that we saw at Plymouth.

My learning curve was vertical. This was the first time I had worked in a multidisciplinary management team. And what a team! The newly-appointed Chief Executive was Peter Griffiths, who subsequently became Deputy Chief Executive for the Management Executive at the Department of Health; Jo Plant, the Chief Nursing Officer, who continued to support and mentor me; Professor Elaine Murphy, Head of Psychiatric Services, who was the first female professor of psychiatry; and Roger Lewis, Consultant Physician in charge of geriatric services (as they were called then). A consultant from the King's Fund, Richard Brazil, was brought in to find ways of exploiting the social security benefits system to pay for the new housing arrangements for people discharged from the mental handicap hospital. Nan Carle, the lead for the mental handicap developments, introduced the concept of 'normalisation' as the driver for these services. The whole place buzzed with new ideas and enthusiasm for their implementation.

We had to fight for most things at St Olave's, for example, to get carpets on the floor as carpets were considered 'not suitable for incontinent old people'. We also fought for keys for the residents' own rooms as we wanted to enable residents' privacy and sense of ownership, but this plan was vehemently opposed by the Fire Department. We did a lot of work to try to establish the ideal size of such a home, which would be small enough to be 'homely' yet large enough to be economically viable. St Olave's Nursing Home finally opened in 1987, soon after I had left, only to be later sold off to the private sector in line with the total privatisation of care homes which took place during the 1990s.

West Lambeth 1986–8

When the project money ran out and the new management arrangements continued to be implemented, I had to move. I was wondering what to do when I had a visit from the two heads of community nursing services – health visiting and district nursing – in the neighbouring West Lambeth (St Thomas') Health District. There too the management arrangements were being restructured, the community services were being reorganised, and their two posts were being combined into one. I assumed that they were coming to see me in my RCN role to seek help in protecting their personal positions, but that was not the issue. They were both taking early retirement. What they wanted, they said, was 'someone like you' to protect the community nursing services that they had built up. They wanted me to apply for the new post of Director of Community Nursing Services in their restructured Community Unit. Having no management experience, I said they were mad. Then about a week later I had a telephone call from Caroline Langridge, the newly-appointed Unit General Manager, asking me to apply.

One of the results of the Griffiths Report from which I personally benefited was that the old hierarchical system of nurse management completely disappeared. One of the reasons why I had been unsuccessful in my efforts to obtain a management post in Berkshire was that because of my 'time out' bringing up my children I did not have the 'right' qualifications or previous experience. For example, for some reason one requirement was to be a qualified health visitor fieldwork instructor, but the training for this qualification was not open to part timers like me so I did not have it. Now, under the new philosophy, all sorts of people were being brought in as NHS managers – army generals, businessmen, entrepreneurs, and others without traditional NHS management careers. Caroline herself had never been a NHS manager, but she had achieved a reputation as Chair of the Lambeth Community Health Council, which itself had achieved considerable notoriety.

I reminded her that I had no management experience. 'Doesn't matter,' she said. 'What if I tell you that my two top priorities for my first year in post are to introduce Cumberlege neighbourhood nursing teams and nurse practitioners in primary care?' That bait did the trick: these were the two issues on which I had been working with Ainna Fawcett-Henesy and Julia Cumberlege herself over the past year, and these were the two key recommendations of the Cumberlege Report that we most wanted to see implemented. I applied, and was appointed.

West Lambeth also was a hotbed of revolutionary new ideas. My base was at the South Western Hospital in Brixton, an old smallpox hospital that, apart from a specialist ward for people on 'iron lung' ventilators as a result of the polio epidemics of the 1940s, catered for long-stay elderly patients and formed part of the community unit. We called it 'the Best Western'.

I was fortunate to have an inspirational nurse manager, Anne Jones, who was responsible for the day-to-day management of the hospital. Building on my experience of the NHS nursing home project at St Olave's, I shared her vision of how care of older people should be, and it was her commitment and enthusiasm for this field of nursing that fired my own later work in this area. She had already achieved miracles, but within the District her contribution, like the care of older people in general, was not recognised nor valued. In the most unprepossessing environment of a Victorian fever hospital, she had tried to make a home-from-home. She had divided the large open wards into individual spaces by means of 'walls' for which patients chose their own wallpaper, she had converted an unused ward into a pub/café area that could be used as a public area where patients and relatives could enjoy a drink together, she had introduced ward housekeepers, and she had developed one of the first 'activities' teams, led by a state-enrolled nurse called Theresa Briscoe. Theresa went on to become the first winner of the *Nursing Standard*'s Nurse of the Year award, and wrote a guidebook to help nurses working with older people to develop their own activity programmes.

The first thing we did was to draw up a statement of our values and beliefs about continuing care services for elderly people. We specified our goal as: 'To enable elderly people who can no longer continue to live independently in the community to live as full and worthwhile a life as possible, maintaining as far as is possible their independence, dignity and self-determination; and to ensure that each is enabled, when life is completed, to die peacefully and with dignity.' We specified our philosophy as follows:

The Continuing Care Services reflect the following beliefs and values:

1. *The patient is central to the services provided; their needs are the reason for and the major determinant of all services.*
2. *Each patient is a unique human being; we acknowledge each person's life experience and personal worth and his/her rights to dignity, privacy and self-determination.*
3. *The quality of life in old age, as at other times, depends upon being able to achieve one's full potential as a human being. This implies the satisfaction not only of basic physical needs but also of emotional, social, and spiritual needs, and opportunities for social and recreational activities and for the enjoyment of satisfying relationships with other people.*
4. *The quality of life of the elderly person in hospital depends directly upon the quality of the environment and the care provided. The quality of care reflects the collective commitment and expertise of the multi-disciplinary hospital team. No one profession has the monopoly of expertise and the contribution of each person is crucial to the care provided by the whole team.*
5. *Elderly people receiving long-term care in hospital have a right to parity of treatment and care with other hospital patients, including access to the full range of diagnostic and therapeutic services designed to treat illness and promote recovery.*
6. *The provision of care is a partnership between the patient and his/her carers, including his/her family. Each patient has the right to participate in the planning and management of his/her own care and to refuse care if s/he wishes.*

It is salutary to reflect that that was written in January 1988, nearly 30 years ago. We are still struggling to achieve it today.

There are those who criticise, or even ridicule, the writing of such mission statements or philosophies, but my experience is that people need a vision to hang on to, especially when the going is tough, as it certainly was for nursing in West Lambeth at that time. My management/leadership style has always been to create the vision, disseminate and share it, and implement it through working with stakeholders bottom-up in groups such as taskforces and committees. So the next thing we did was to write a strategy for implementing these values, which we called 'Nursing 1990', and to establish a Nursing 1990 Group composed of all the ward sisters, night sisters, and sisters from the two day units, which met monthly and acted as a vehicle for the discussion of developmental ideas, for training, and as a professional peer support group. We committed ourselves to changing the philosophy of caring for older people from the old 'custodial/warehousing' model to one that reflected individualised care based on individually assessed needs.

I was also responsible for the Lambeth Community Care Centre, although day-to-day management was vested in the small multidisciplinary centre management team (senior nurse, administrator, therapist, GP and centre advisory group chairperson) under the expert leadership of the senior nurse, Sheila Woodward. It was a beautifully designed purpose-built building with 20 beds, 35 day places, physiotherapy, occupational therapy, speech therapy, dental services, social workers, dietician, chiropodist, general surgery outpatients, and facilities for education, groups, local community and voluntary organisations. Medical care was provided by contracted GPs. Patients came from two local London boroughs, Lambeth and Southwark, and three health authorities: West Lambeth, Lewisham, and North Southwark and Camberwell. In 1988 it was providing just the kind of care that is today aspired to as 'best practice' but is still rarely found. The individual patient was in charge of his/her own care, an integral part of the team of nurse, therapist(s) and GP, and was involved in agreeing problem lists, setting objectives and managing his/her care, including being responsible for his/her own medication. Records were open to patients and used centrally by all carers, writing within a problem-orientated framework. All patients had a key worker or special nurse who was responsible for coordinating care with the patient and other members of the primary health care team. On the ward this was usually a nurse or sometimes a therapist. In the day unit the worker currently most involved would take on this role. There was always a named carer when the key worker was off duty to ensure clear lines of accountability and communication, particularly with the patient.

My next task was to re-organise the community nurses into neighbourhood nursing teams as recommended in the Cumberlege Report. Cumberlege had (rightly in my view) argued that district nurses, health visitors, school nurses, and practice nurses were stuck in the rut of practising and being managed in separate uni-disciplinary silos, and she recommended that they should be brought together into multidisciplinary neighbourhood nursing teams under a single manager serving a geographically-defined population. The neighbourhood nurse manager might come from any of the three main disciplines but would manage all of them together. The proposal was not popular, especially among GPs, who focused their criticism on the recommendation that practice nurses, who were employed by them and not by the district health authority as health visitors and district nurses were, should be integrated into the new teams. The challenge for me, and the task specifically required by the unit general manager, was not only to identify, appoint and train nurses who could undertake this new role, but also to persuade fieldworkers to accept managers from a different discipline. I was able to identify good potential leaders from among the existing staff, but the key to success was the huge effort we put into communication, training and team development.

At this time few practices within the District employed practice nurses, but there was one group practice that was well organised and keen on the idea of the nurse practitioner. For this reason I appointed Barbara Stillwell to work there as the first NHS-employed nurse practitioner. Barbara had almost single-handedly developed the role in primary care in the UK, having undertaken training at the University of North Carolina (Chapel Hill) in the USA, where the role was well developed. She had worked with us as part of the RCN team that had developed the proposal included in the Cumberlege Review. Barbara later developed the first nurse practitioner training programme at the RCN.

Within 18 months I had achieved my two main tasks. I had a wonderful team of nurses and we were making progress towards our goals. However, the introduction of general management was already creating problems for nursing, and in particular for me. Once again my post was overtaken by management restructuring. Sir Roy had never recommended that general management should be used below the level of the unit (the second level in a District), and the 1985 Department of Health Circular on the implementation of general management specifically stated: 'There can be no sustainable improvement at unit level if it does not rest upon the fullest involvement and commitment of all the professions concerned with the delivery of health care, particularly all doctors and nurses.' Caroline, however, wanted to implement it right down to field level. Whereas in the acute unit and the mental health unit full responsibility for the nursing function was delegated by the unit general manager to a director of nursing services, in the restructured community unit the managerial responsibility (the budget and management of staff, including nurses) became the responsibility of locality managers, who in turn were managed by service managers, none of whom had a clinical background; my role as Director of Nursing Services was reduced to an advisory function. The neighbourhood nurse managers became accountable to the locality managers, and I found myself managed by and accountable to a service manager who had little understanding of and no sympathy with nursing. I would not have minded, were it not that she would frequently and with obvious relish remind me with the words: 'Thank you June for your advice, but you must realise that I am now the manager.' The last straw was when she decided to reduce staffing numbers on the wards at South Western and I was powerless to prevent it. Several of the senior nurses left and their posts remained vacant. After I resigned there were no immediate plans to replace me. My last few weeks were spent trying, together with the remaining senior nurses, to establish some systems for maintaining the nursing function until a successor could be appointed. Fortunately, soon after I left the Community Unit was restructured again. Caroline moved to the Department of Health and Ray Rowden became the unit's Chief Executive. Ray abolished the locality managers and kept the neighbourhood managers, all nurses, who reported directly to the new Director of Community Services, Jane Schofield, as they had in the beginning to me.

Once again, although I knew I would have to move on, I was not sure what I should move to. Meanwhile general management systems were being implemented everywhere. One result of this was that at district level chief nursing officer posts were changing to chief nursing adviser posts, just as was happening at unit level. Moreover, whereas under the old system nurse management posts did not vary much from place to place, now they varied enormously according to the wishes of the individual chief executives. Many chief nursing officers were taking on new responsibilities, such as quality assurance. I wondered whether this was the kind of post that Malcolm Ross had been thinking of and thought that with some more information and management training I might be ready to apply. When I saw posts advertised I sent for details to find out what the posts were like and how I might prepare myself. Among the jobs I requested details for was one at Harrow Health Authority. I thought it looked interesting, read it, and then set it aside

Harrow 1988–90

One Friday evening some weeks later I was preparing to leave my office to go away with an old nursing friend, Jean Cubbin, for a weekend city break to Amsterdam. We had planned to meet at Liverpool Street station, so I had my suitcase and my casual clothes with me, planning to go straight from my office. I was just changing when the telephone rang. The voice at the other end said: 'I sent you some details about a post a few weeks ago but I haven't heard from you since.' It was Alan Langlands, the Chief Executive/District General Manager of Harrow Health Authority. The conversation went as follows:

*Me: 'No. Well I was very interested in the details, but I don't think I yet have
the experience you need so I didn't apply.'
Alan: Well, I'd really like you to apply.'
Me: 'But I'm just going to Amsterdam.'
Alan: 'Can we meet to discuss it?'
Me: 'I'm just going to Amsterdam.'
Alan: 'Well the interviews are next Thursday. We're interviewing for several
posts. Can we meet some time before then?'*

Finally we agreed to meet at the only time and place compatible with both
our diaries – at 6 o'clock on the following Monday at the headquarters of the
Regional Health Authority, which was next door to Paddington Station from
where I normally caught the train home.

Jean and I took the overnight ferry, spent Saturday and Sunday
sightseeing, caught the overnight ferry back on Sunday, and I worked a full
day on Monday before meeting Alan as planned at 6pm. I was so tired that I
remember very little about the meeting. When I got home I discussed it with
Roger, who said: 'Well if you're interested in that kind of post, it's a good
opportunity to find out more, so go on Thursday and see what you can find
out.' And so I went. The interview was an all-day affair – presentations about
the district, a 'trial by sherry' attended by members of the health authority,
senior staff of all disciplines, and candidates for the two jobs (heads of
human resources and nursing) to which appointments were to be made, as
well as individual interviews. I liked what I saw, but I did not expect to hear
anything further. Within a week I was offered the post of Chief Nursing
Adviser, and I accepted.

My first day in post coincided with the meeting of the District
Management Team at which the main agenda item was preparation for the
forthcoming meeting of the Health Authority. I had a special interest in this
because until now I had always been at the other side of the table – as nurse
member of the Area Health Authority in Berkshire in the 70s and more
recently in Oxfordshire. So I was quite taken aback when over coffee as we
waited for the meeting to start, one member of the team said: 'Well what are
we going to tell the buggers this time, because we sure can't tell them the
truth!' Such was my naivety.

Alan Langlands was the best boss I ever had. Some years later, in an
interview for one of the health journals, he said: 'Leadership comes in
more forms than just the macho, riding-a-white-charger variety. Leadership

in the health service is about something more subtle than that. It's about influencing skills, about being able to understand the problems of working across professional boundaries, about releasing creative energy within organisations.' He knew what he wanted, and he got it, but always through developing and empowering people, never through the bullying, controlling styles that I have experienced elsewhere. Although his first commitment was always to patients, he really cared about his staff: on Fridays at about 6pm he would walk round the team members' offices, saying 'Go home' to each one. I was never made to feel that I was 'only' an adviser. And whatever his final decision, he always listened.

On the first anniversary of taking up post, I took him a bottle of wine and a card with the message: 'Thank you for taking the risk.' His reply was: 'I don't know how to tell you this, June, but I'm leaving Harrow.' Disenchanted with the reforms, and especially the purchaser–provider split, he left to set up a European consultancy arm for the multinational company Towers Perrin. It was not long before he was called back to take over at regional level, however, when the Regional General Manager fell ill. Later he was to become head of the NHS as a whole.

At the time Alan left, the planned service reorganisation was so close that the Department of Health refused to sanction the appointment of a new District General Manager and instead seconded an under-secretary in the Department of Health, the second-in-charge of their Finance Directorate, John James, to fill the vacancy. At first John was a pleasure to work with. As a high-flying civil servant, his IQ was at least 10 points higher than I had experienced anywhere else in the NHS. The challenge was fun and I think he thought so too. When I left he wrote: 'All of us will miss your lively and distinctive contribution to our deliberations, and I personally will miss the intellectual stimulus that you constantly gave.' Of course, another interpretation of that might be: 'Thank goodness for that. Now I can get on with things the way I want to!'

The most urgent task was to deal with the 'clinical grading' appeals. As the culmination of the pay campaigns of the 1980s, the introduction of a new pay system for nurses with a grading scale based on clearly specified job descriptions was introduced. At first nurses were optimistic that at last they would get appropriate recognition and reward for their clinical skills. They were to be disappointed. Cash limits were imposed so that district health authorities and trust boards were told how many posts they could have at each grade. Appeals were inevitable, and hearing them dominated the agendas of chief nurses and the RCN for the next 5 years. The good news was the requirement that every nurse should in future have a written job description that adequately described his/her knowledge and skills. The bad news was the content that the job descriptions and the information presented in the appeals revealed – routinised and task-oriented approaches to patient care, fragmentation of responsibility, confusion about professional accountability, and nurses who had been in the same job for 20 years without any professional development or updating. I wept for the unrealised potential and committed myself to trying to do something about it.

Developing practice

In persuading me to apply, Alan had told me that he wanted a nurse who 'burned for' and really knew about nursing, and I had no doubts about my ability in that area but was very anxious about my lack of orthodox management experience. The vision that had drawn me to Harrow in the first place was the possibility of developing Harrow as a centre of excellence in nursing rather like I was seeing in Oxfordshire, where I was still nurse member of the Health Authority. I hoped to do this through things like clinical practice development, creating a nursing development unit similar to the one at Burford, and recreating the nursing research unit at Northwick Park Hospital. I had lots of ideas and it was a real blow to discover that far from sharing my excitement about nursing, once again others saw these things as a threat to general management within the units.

Using my experience in West Lambeth, one of the first things I did was to start working with the Nursing Advisory Committee to develop a statement of our vision and values. It was called 'Nursing in Harrow', and we prepared it as a poster to put on the noticeboard of every ward and health centre throughout the District, and as a little laminated card that every nurse could carry in his or her pocket. The content was very similar to what I had developed in West Lambeth, but even more important was the way in which I was able to use the Nursing Advisory Committee as a vehicle to provide professional development, training, and support during a period when nursing was continually being threatened within the developing general management structures.

Our next initiative was to start work on developing quality assurance for nursing. I had been involved in quality assurance and standards in nursing since the 1970s and had been a member of the RCN Working Party on Standards of Care, which had produced the two documents *Standards of Care* (1980) and *Towards Standards* (1981). I had taken these ideas to my job as Senior Nurse (Research) in Berkshire in 1983, where with Helen

Kendall I had established what became the RCN's Dynamic Standard Setting System (DySSy). The Nursing Quality Group was established as a subgroup of the Nursing Advisory Committee. It was just at the time that medical audit was becoming popular, but we believed that, to be useful, the concept had to be extended to cover all disciplines including nursing. The Nursing Quality Group became the Nursing Quality and Audit Committee, chaired by Paula Crouch. We developed question and answer seminars and facilitators' training sessions and invited paramedics and therapists to join us.

Managing nursing education

My main management responsibility was nursing education. Traditionally, final responsibility for a district's school of nursing rested with the chief nursing officer, but this responsibility was always fully delegated to a director of nursing education. In the week before I arrived at Harrow, the Director of Nursing Education and the Assistant Director for Pre-registration Education had both left. Owing to changes in nursing education (the changes in funding and the introduction of the new Project 2000 programmes), these two posts were immediately frozen and I found myself directly managing a School of Nursing whose staff would be the first to admit there were problems. Moreover, the School of Nursing was due to be amalgamated with the Brent and Harrow School of Midwifery at the other end of the Northwick Park campus. In addition to this, the Regional Health Authority was promoting the amalgamation of these two schools with St Mary's (Paddington) School of Midwifery and St Mary's School of Nursing, the latter being one of the pilot sites for the introduction of Project 2000. The well-known and charismatic Director of Nursing Education at St Mary's, Stanley Holder, had also just retired. There was a huge transition to be managed and a dearth of people to see it through while maintaining the programmes currently in place for students already in training. The target was to establish a new Harrow and Parkside College of Nursing and Midwifery, serving both Harrow and Parkside Health Authorities, by 1 April 1990.

Preparatory tasks included consolidating the multiple nursing revenue budgets of the two district health authorities, the separate midwifery education (including student salaries) budget, the central funding channelled through the Regional Health Authority for teachers' salaries, trust funds, and new moneys being made available for the introduction of Project 2000. There had to be changes in the contracts of employment of staff and students, including differences in London weighting. There were eight sites to be managed. A principal for the new College would need to be appointed and a management structure developed. A steering group was established, composed of the chief nursing advisors and the directors of personnel of both health authorities. This was later extended by inclusion of the finance directors and Harrow's District General Manager John James, and became a transition board chaired by Barbara Young, Parkside's District General Manager. Of all these people, only the two chief nursing advisors had any previous knowledge or experience of nursing education – and my experience was limited, to say the least.

I was assisted and supported by two wonderful people. One was Bob Hancock, the only remaining Assistant Director of Nursing Education at the Brent and Harrow School. Bob was originally responsible for post-registration education but now took over the management of the whole school; despite stepping up, however, his appointment as Director of Nursing Education was vetoed by the Regional Health Authority. The other person was Neslyn Watson-Druee, whom I appointed as my Project 2000 Project Officer. I appointed Ursula Cowell, formerly Director of Nurse Education at the St Thomas' Nightingale School of Nursing, as Principal of the new combined School.

The next phase of the general management revolution, in which Harrow was to be one of the flagships, was the introduction of clinical directorates. This was part of the attempt to engage doctors, the biggest spenders of health care resources, in resource management and to make them accountable for their expenditure. The plan was to follow the organisational model developed at Johns Hopkins Hospital, Baltimore, USA, which was being heavily promoted by the Department of Health and King's Fund, which had seconded a consultant to Harrow to help implement the project. Each clinical field was to form a managerial unit headed by a physician who held the budget for the directorate's service and was accountable for the directorate's functioning, budgetary control, and management of staff (including nurses), equipment and supplies. All of the clinical directors were to be members of the management board, alongside functional directors such as the Director of Finance and Director of Human Resources. The problem for nursing was that there was no place for a nurse on the management board. The most senior nurse in the organisation would be the most senior nurse – probably a ward sister – within each directorate, who would be accountable to the clinical director. Once again nursing would be demoted to the third level down in the management structure, and there would be no mechanism for achieving whole-organisation nursing policy, professional leadership or accountability.

I knew from my contacts in the USA that there every hospital had a vice president for nursing who was an influential member of the board and who provided professional leadership for the nursing staff. I therefore organised a study visit for our management team to visit Johns Hopkins and some other hospitals in Baltimore, New York and Washington to find out how things worked. The day before we visited Johns Hopkins we visited the Maryland Medical Centre next door, where we found a nursing management team who had moved there from the Johns Hopkins Hospital because they had found that the latter's arrangements did not work. At the Johns Hopkins Hospital the following day, the Chief Executive himself told us that the system was unique to Johns Hopkins and had been developed to meet its specific needs as a hospital whose main purpose was teaching and research rather than the delivery of healthcare. (All patients were required to consent to participate in a research programme as a condition of treatment.) The Chief Executive Officer of one of the other hospitals we visited described it as 'a collection of competing fiefdoms'.

While we were away, *The Times* published an editorial supporting the changes. In the issue of 7 July 1990, my response was published.

Sir,

Fresh off the plane from the USA on June 30th, I read your editorial 'A healthier service'. [...] At every one of the seven hospitals we visited in Baltimore, Washington and New York people were amazed and appalled at proposals which they identified as the route from which they were trying to escape. We had hoped to find, and to be able to learn from, financial and information systems which could support the costing and pricing requirements of our new contracting environment. Instead we found huge investment (from which, they said, only the computer vendors and the management consultants benefited) in systems which merely 'fed the beast' of reimbursement systems and federal requirements, and in an army of financial reviewers, utilisation reviewers and highly paid coders. We found that the decentralised management system of clinical directorates which has been developed at Johns Hopkins Hospital [...] has major problems in its hospital of origin and does not appear to have been replicated anywhere else in the States. We found cut-throat competition between hospitals. [...] We found that purchasing authorities, far from demanding improvements in quality, were negotiating discount deals with providers on the basis of volume. In New York in particular we saw casualty departments which resembled cattle markets, with sick people waiting for admission to a ward for up to 72 hours on trolleys lined up edge to edge in corridors. We also saw some good things which, paradoxically are not part of our NHS proposals: consumer protection based on a patient's Bill of Rights..., the right [for patients] to see their medical record and access to each individual doctor's credentials, quality assurance systems based on a accreditation (a concept which has been rejected by our secretary of state), value accorded to nursing at the level not only of direct patient care but of corporate policy making in posts which are being discontinued in the NHS, major investment in nursing education.... The administration costs of American hospitals were estimated for us at 23% compared with our 5%.

The final paragraph read: 'Since Kenneth Clarke, the Secretary of State, has said "It will happen", no doubt it will, and it will be difficult for any alternative government to undo, but let us not deceive ourselves that it will produce better value for money or a service in which the quality of care is the primary concern.' More than 20 years on, time has proved me right.

To prepare for the coming reorganisation, we were required to undergo a series of 'management games' based on scenarios of what it would be like to work in the new order. For one game we were divided into three teams – one purchaser and two providers. We were allowed to choose which team we joined, and since, as a result of my health visiting background, I was attracted by the idea of purchasing services based on epidemiological data and assessment of the community's needs, I joined the purchasing team. When we started at 8.30am, each team (in separate rooms) was given relevant data on which to decide its strategies for providing services to the defined community. The two providers were in competition with each other to capture the purchaser's contracts. In the purchasing team we were quite clear that we must put quality at least as high as cost, and we planned accordingly. During our deliberations a messenger came several times with new information, for example that Provider A could undertake more hip replacements at lower unit cost if the purchaser would agree to contract for some other service that the provider wanted to provide. We worked hard until about 10.30am, when we stopped for coffee. Over coffee I suddenly realised that we in the purchasing team had changed our tactics from our original plans, and were now placing contracts almost exclusively on the basis of lowest cost. It was just what our American colleagues had told us, and I began to feel very uncomfortable about what the forthcoming reorganisation might mean.

A few weeks later I had a meeting of my ward sisters, who had been discussing ways of ensuring that the about-to-be-introduced medical audit included nursing. They were a great bunch of people, and I came out as high as a kite with enthusiasm about what they were planning. In the corridor I bumped into John James, and was bursting to tell him about it, but he said: 'Don't bother about that now, I've just been walking the corridors of the hospital; we have nearly 2 miles of potential advertising space, and it's going to be your job to sell it!' My heart fell into my boots. That was not what I had come into nursing for. I knew in that instant that although I loved the challenge of change, I could not cope with the cognitive dissonance between what would be expected of me in the new order and my deep-seated values about nursing and patient care. I would have to go and find another job.

A new challenge

I was again unsure what job to apply for next. Then, at a dinner that was held for the chief nurses of the North West Thames region, the buzz of conversation that followed guest speaker Catherine McLaughlin was all about the changes. Most of my colleagues were planning to take early retirement, for which a generous package had been negotiated, but at 48 years I was just too young to be eligible. I shared my worries with Judith Sears, Chief Nurse to Barnet Health Authority, who was sitting next to me. She thought for a moment and then said: 'I know just the job for you.' She proceeded to tell me about the work she had been doing with Middlesex Polytechnic to establish a new degree-level nursing programme that, it was hoped, would attract high-flying nurses to work for the local health authorities. The plan was that the new school would appoint staff who would teach all the '-ologies', Barnet School of Nursing would provide all the clinical content and Barnet Health Authority the clinical placements. 'But they need a Head of School,' she said, 'someone to lead it, someone like you.'

For 30 years I had resolved to have nothing to do with nursing education, which I regarded as a rigid repressive training and nothing like the education I thought nurses ought to have. I believed training should be in a university setting and at degree level – a view not widely shared in the profession. My only educational experience at that time was as a student and through my work in Harrow, but Judith persisted. She reminded me of the baptism of fire I had just experienced in my role as the person responsible for nursing education in Harrow. Since I had survived that, she pointed out, I knew plenty about nursing education. And since the Polytechnic was about to become a university, they needed people with academic as well as nursing credibility. I was one of very few nurses with a PhD. At her insistence I agreed to apply, and was appointed.

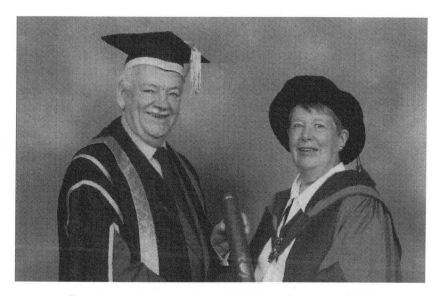

Receiving an honorary degree, Middlesex University, 1994

CHAPTER 5: NURSING EDUCATION: MIDDLESEX UNIVERSITY

Under the headline 'Nurses' leader heads Poly's new Health Care Studies School', North Circular, the Middlesex Polytechnic newspaper reported:

One of the country's leading nurses, Dr June Clark, has been appointed head of the polytechnic's new school of Health Care Studies, with the title of Professor. The dean of the faculty of Social Science, Professor Edmund Penning-Rowsell, said: 'Dr Clark is one of the most distinguished nurses in the country. We are very pleased that she is joining us'. Dr Clark told North Circular that she was very excited at the idea of developing the new school. 'The partnership between the polytechnic and the five local health authorities provides an opportunity to bring together academic excellence with a wealth of clinical excellence and expertise.'

And the idea was exciting. The 'pull factor' was the opportunity to actually implement ideas that I had been promoting for 30 years but never been in a position to action. The Polytechnic, which was about to become one of the 'new universities', had a business plan that included rapid expansion in nursing student numbers from 49 to 340, supported by a growth in staffing numbers from 4.4 to 17 full-time equivalents by the 1993–4 academic year. Even without the changes planned for the following few years, the plan was hopelessly over-ambitious. Despite this, we were not deterred.

The School was formally launched in November 1990 as part of Middlesex's contribution to National Polytechnics Week, which celebrated the 21st anniversary of the establishment of the polytechnic. I gave a public lecture before an audience of around 150 invited guests, the title of which, 'On these rocks...' (taken from Margretta Styles' 'A Biblical Fable on Our Origins', *On Nursing: Toward a New Endowment*), was chosen to set out the values and aspirations of the new School:

> *In the beginning God created nursing.*
> *He (or she) said:*
> *I will take a solid simple significant system of education,*
> *And an adequate applicable base of clinical research,*
> *And on these rocks,*
> *I will build my greatest gift to Mankind – nursing practice.*
> *On the seventh day, He threw up his hands,*
> *And he has left it up to us.*

The foundation (the rocks) on which the School was to be built was the integration between education, research and clinical practice, and a commitment to bridge the 'theory–practice divide' in nursing. This core value, which I had promoted throughout my career, was the basis for the new degree in nursing, for the partnerships between the University and the NHS-based Schools of Nursing, and for the establishment of the Middlesex Academic Nursing Units.

I took up my post as Head of the new School of Health Care Studies in September 1990. It could not have chosen a worse time to be created as we were caught up in the changes to nursing education proposed as a result of Project 2000 and the Thatcherite reforms of the NHS. What I had experienced at Harrow was just a taster. Changes in the regional health authorities' strategies for nursing education led to the amalgamation of schools of nursing to form new colleges. District health authorities merged or changed their boundaries. Most seriously, the NHS and Community Care Act 1990 removed the responsibility and the financial resources for nursing education from the district health authorities and established the principle that employers – the new NHS trusts and other 'provider units' – should be responsible for nursing education on the basis of contracts with education providers. As a result, the original partners were no longer in a position to deliver their original agreements. The North West Thames Region was the first to put nursing education out to tender, and Barnet School of Nursing did not win the contract. Middlesex therefore withdrew from its plans to merge, the Barnet School of Nursing was wiped out, and its staff members were made redundant. As part of the reorganisation that followed the government White Paper *Working with Patients, Working Paper 10* – which dealt with the education and training implications of the NHS reforms – referred only briefly to undergraduate nursing courses, which were still comparatively rare: it assumed a 'status quo' for existing undergraduate courses and proposed to discuss with the Universities Funding Council the funding arrangement for future courses. For Middlesex, the timing of these arrangements was disastrous. It did not have an 'existing' course and the start of the new BA nursing programme was too imminent to await arrangements for 'new' courses. Guidance on the implementation of the proposals was delayed, and the uncertainty of funding was hugely detrimental to the development of the School.

Moreover, the government having suddenly pulled back on its support for polytechnics, this period coincided with a period of severe financial restraint within Middlesex Polytechnic. The ambitious business plan was abandoned. The 'old' Principal, who had stayed on past retirement age to see in the implementation of plans in which he had played a key role, left and was replaced by new Vice-Chancellor, David Melville, who had a totally different agenda with totally different priorities.

The team

My first task was to appoint some staff. In April 1991 Dr Janet Higgins and Dr Kevin Gournay joined my team. I chose Janet as my deputy because as a physician she had been involved for several years in medical education, partly in the polytechnic sector, and I thought she would compensate for my lack of experience in this field. Kevin was qualified both as a psychiatric and a learning disabilities nurse. He had a PhD and a passion for research – a very rare set of qualifications. I was warned not to appoint him because he was a 'wild card', but that was exactly what I wanted, and over the next year or so he more than justified my hopes. Kevin went on to become the first Professor of Psychiatric Nursing at the Maudsley Hospital in London. While at Middlesex he was responsible for developing the School's research programme and the mental health branch of the nursing degree. Dr Elizabeth Clark, a psychologist with considerable experience in teaching nurses and in distance learning (which, it was expected, would be developed as part of the strategy for managing the proposed great expansion in student numbers), was appointed at the same time. I came to rely very heavily on her enormous wisdom as time went on.

Thus all four of us held doctorates, which must have been a first for any school of nursing in the country. It was exactly what the university wanted but it was not enough for the English National Board, who at the final stage of the validation of the nursing programme announced that it could not approve the programme because none of us held the sister tutor's diploma and were thus not competent to teach nurses. At the last minute I therefore had to appoint a registered nurse tutor. Barbara Shailer joined us 8 weeks before the course was to begin.

Practical issues

My 'office' (in anticipation of the promised new building) was a windowless cubby-hole in a building on an industrial estate in Enfield. The journey from home was a nightmare: 62 miles door-to-door, but entirely on the M4 and the M25; to minimise traffic delays I left home early and arrived home late. I had an excellent secretary, Kate Jarvis, who had moved from another part of the Polytechnic and thus knew the organisation. I also had a cardboard box containing the programmes and plans for the programme. Computerisation was still to come. When the first 49 students arrived, it was to a school without adequate teaching equipment or accommodation, to a course whose leader had been in post for only 8 weeks, and to a programme of five modules in the first semester, all of which were being taught for the first time. We learned together, however, and some of that cohort remained in contact with me until long after I had left Middlesex.

I was particularly keen to have a professorial nursing unit. This combined two ideas that were already well-established and familiar but had never, as far as I knew, been combined – the medical professorial units found in teaching hospitals where, for example, the Professor of Surgery had his or her own wards where he or she saw patients and focused on his or her own research, and the nursing development units that had been established over the previous decade supported by the King's Fund, in places such as Oxfordshire and Tameside, without specific academic links. I wanted a unit where I could undertake clinical practice and focus my own and the School's research programme.

I found such a place at Colindale Hospital, a small Victorian fever hospital then used for rehabilitation and the long-term care of older people. I have always argued, and still do argue, that it is in the care of older people that 'real' nursing can be found, and where nursing can really make a difference. Nurse Manager Rose Harte continued to manage the unit, and I appointed a young man as the Clinical Practice Development Nurse. This role is now fairly common but in those days was rare. I tried to work one shift a week, usually arriving after work in the university. I worked on the ward until about 11pm, stayed overnight in the Nurses' Home, worked on the ward again for a few hours the following morning, and then returned to the university for the rest of the day. It was not easy, but the biggest problem was persuading the ward staff that, in spite of being a professor, my level of competence in clinical nursing was no greater than that of any other basic-grade staff nurse!

At this time I was also President of the RCN, and one of my presidential duties was to dine with the presidents of the other Royal Colleges. The pattern of conversation was always the same – so much so that after the first few occasions I deliberately pursued it as a game. Over sherry there would be introductions, followed by talk about the weather or current events until we went in for dinner. In the dining room, table places were labelled with our names and titles – in my case Professor June Clark (I was not yet a dame). My neighbour would look across at my place card and say in a surprised tone: 'Oh I didn't know you had professors of nursing.' I would respond: 'Oh yes, there are quite a few of us now that nursing education is moving into the universities.' There would be congratulations followed by something along the lines of: 'I'm so pleased that you girls [sic] are getting some recognition at last. But I do think it's sad that as soon as you move up the scale you give up nursing patients.' I explained that although difficult, I had a professorial nursing unit where I worked one shift a week. At this point the other person would nearly disappear under the table in shock. Then after a short pause I would be asked where my Unit was, with the expectation that it would be in one of the famous London teaching hospitals. I would say: 'It's at Colindale Hospital, which is a small facility for long-term care of older people.' At this point the person would really disappear under the table, and I would go for the jugular. 'Yes I love it. It's so much more interesting than medicine. Matter of fact I was working with an old lady this morning. Ninety years old, lives on her own, never been in a hospital before, totally independent until a couple of weeks ago when she fell and fractured her femur. You boys [sic] did a good job of your bit – I think that's the easy bit – and then you just passed her over to us. Thanks to you she should be able to stand and walk, but she can't because she's terrified. She thinks it's all over, she's not eating or drinking, and she's a bit confused. But so would I be if I'd never been in hospital before and then got shunted from ward to ward for a week and then moved to a completely different place. Nobody has explained what's happening to her. And then – terrible thing – last night she couldn't get out of bed and there was no one to help her and she wet the bed. She was devastated. I think that sorting out all those problems in ways that suit her and preserve her dignity and autonomy are a tremendous intellectual challenge. I also got enormous job satisfaction from building a relationship with her. That's why I find nursing so challenging.'

I played this 'game' on several occasions, until on the fourth or fifth occasion my neighbour said: 'Hmm. That's really interesting. I've never heard it put that way before. Could you do me 1000 words by next Friday?' It was Richard Smith, then Editor of the *British Medical Journal*. My 1000 words appeared as an editorial in the *BMJ* of 17 August 1991 under the strap-line 'Nursing: an intellectual activity'.

It was not the first time I had written about this idea. Back in 1986 I had a piece published in the *Nursing Times* entitled 'Free from the straitjacket', which argued:

There are, broadly speaking, two ways of looking at nursing, and which of the two you choose determine your whole perspective on the nursing world.... The first way of looking at nursing sees it as a collection of tasks, some requiring more skill than others, whose function is to support the medical function of treating disease. Nursing is seen as a craft rather than a profession. The second, and quite different perspective sees nursing as a particular kind of interaction [between a professional and a patient] which has certain specific goals distinct from those of medicine and involves particular kinds of activities. These activities depend upon and reflect the thought processes and the decisions which give rise to them, and it is this that distinguishes professional nursing from similar activities performed by unqualified carers. Knowledge is the essential prerequisite for sound decision making, so education as opposed to training, is fundamental.

The *BMJ* article stimulated considerable correspondence in the journal, mainly about nurses who 'got above themselves'. It was reprinted in the *International Nursing Review* (the journal of the ICN) but received no mention in the British nursing press. Sadly, over 20 years on, the NHS and UK nursing are still firmly stuck in the first paradigm.

Achievements

It was tough, very tough. Nevertheless, in my first annual report, covering the period 1990 to 1992, I was able to report the following achievements:

- Validation and two intakes of an innovative programme leading to a BA (Nursing) with registration as a nurse
- Validation and initial intake of a health studies (minor) set within the University's modular degree scheme
- Validation and initial intake of a postgraduate diploma in health care provision
- Establishment of three Middlesex Academic Nursing Units, including the Professorial Nursing Unit at Colindale Hospital
- Establishment of the Middlesex Mental Health Research Unit in Parkside Health Authority
- Development of a programme of multidisciplinary research within the University's Health Research Centre
- Establishment of a Division of Public Health in association with Barnet Health Authority's Department of Public Health
- A programme of consultancy that had generated income in excess of £100 000 (a substantial sum in those days)
- Development of an international network of seven countries within Europe, supported by the EU Erasmus programme, and links with universities in USA.

Not all these initiatives were sustained, but the two of which I was most proud were the Professorial Nursing Unit and the international networking programme. In addition to the student and teacher exchanges, which were the core of the EU Erasmus programmes, I developed and taught a module on international health care, which was replicated by each of our partners so that students who could not travel to another country, for example because of family commitments, could at least interact with students from other countries and learn something about their cultures and health care systems. The essays the students wrote as the assessment for this module were presented in seminars so that everyone could share their learning.

Work in Kazakhstan

One of my most interesting projects came through collaboration with the University's Kazakhstan–UK Centre, which was led by sociologist Greg Andrusz. In 1990, the Soviet Union started to break up and its former constituent republics declared independence one by one. Kazakhstan became independent in 1991. By the end of that year, the Soviet Union ceased to exist, leaving an enormous political, economic and social vacuum behind.

In response, the European Union established the Technical Assistance to the Commonwealth of Independent States, or TACIS, programme. UK Government support was provided through the British Know-How Fund in the form of grants to UK organisations enabling individuals to visit Kazakhstan to provide 'technical advice'. Jane Salvage, then World Health Organization (WHO) Adviser for Nursing and Midwifery at the Regional Office for Europe, was already running leadership development workshops for newly-independent states' nurses in collaboration with the WHO Collaborating Centre at Alma Ata. Virginia Bottomley, Secretary of State for Health, visited Kazakhstan in 1991 to promote the British healthcare system. In 1992 we were successful in getting a contract to run a workshop to help Kazakh politicians and health service managers identify projects to be funded by the British Government to help rebuild their healthcare system.

With Jibek Karagoulova, Head of the WHO Collaborating Centre, Alma Ata, 1993

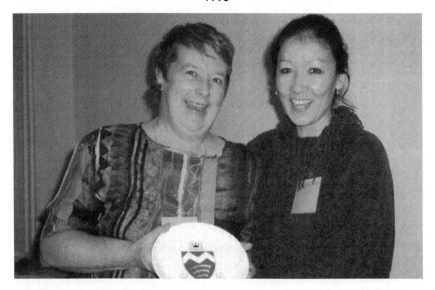

I led a team of health professionals and health service managers including Sir Duncan Nichol, who had recently retired as Director of the NHS, Chris Paine (now Sir Christopher), a consultant oncologist who was also a district chief executive, Steve Collins, a lecturer from the local further education college, and Martin Taylor, a young anthropologist who served as translator and administrative assistant. We were supported by two civil servants from the UK Government and by Dr Jibek Karagoulova, who was Head of the local WHO Collaborating Centre. The challenge of the core task was greatly increased by the organisational and physical challenges resulting from the complete lack of infrastructure and basic facilities such as transport, water, electricity and banks. Without banks, Martin had to carry $50 000 in cash on his person in low-denomination bills to pay the bills. Electricity and hot water were limited to about 4 hours a day. We had to take everything we would need with us, down to the paper and pens.

On the day before the workshop was due to start, a programme of visits to local healthcare facilities was arranged. Chris and I visited the cancer hospital in Alma Ata – the country's showpiece. We were shown around by the Director, who smoked throughout our visit; when challenged by Chris, the Director said that he did not believe that the link between smoking and cancer was yet proven! In the basement the Director proudly showed us his latest acquisition – a large scanner supplied by the French government, still in its wrapping because there was not enough electricity to enable it to be used. As we walked through the basement Chris trod on something that squelched. It was a very-dead rat.

During four visits to Kazakhstan between 1993 and 1995 I visited several other healthcare facilities, including a school of nursing and a TB hospital. It was like taking a step back in time. The facilities and equipment looked rather like those I had experienced back in the early 1960s in the UK. The nurses, dressed in white coats and the typical Russian nurse's cap, which is rather like the UK chef's hat, were clearly operating entirely under medical direction. What shocked me most, though, was the way that the patients were treated. There was no privacy or respect, as highlighted by the way in which individuals were picked out as 'demonstrations' as we went from ward to ward.

Goulnara

On two occasions when I visited Kazakhstan I combined TACIS work with Jane Salvage's WHO leadership development workshops. No one spoke English, so we used local translators. One was Goulnara Beckmukhamedova, who had also acted as translator for the WHO and Jane Salvage's nurse leader workshops, and who became a good friend.

On my first visit to the country in 1993 I travelled with Goulnara, who was returning from a WHO meeting in the UK. We took a British Airways flight to Moscow, then had to get a bus across Moscow from Sheremetyevo International Airport to Domodedovo (domestic) Airport to take an Aeroflot flight to Alma Ata. At Domodedovo we waited a long time for the Aeroflot plane in a cavernous hall with no facilities, and then had to walk across the tarmac carrying our luggage to load it ourselves. Inside, the aircraft was like the troop carriers we see on TV. There were no seat belts. It was an 8-hour journey. Food in the shape of half a chicken and a large piece of bread was offered, but Goulnara warned me not to touch the chicken; fortunately we had our own supply of bottled water. (Thankfully, by the time of our subsequent visits British Airways was running direct flights to Alma Ata.)

I helped Goulnara to leave Kazakhstan with her daughter Camilla, then only 11 years old, to start a new life. Goulnara's one wish was to get Camilla to England so that she could go to an English university. Goulnara had trained as a translator at Moscow University, and while working for the WHO had come top in a highly competitive exam for a post in the BBC Monitoring Centre in Reading (where I lived). The process of getting her and Camilla out of Kazakhstan was much more complicated than getting

With Goulnara, Camilla and Anel, the Mumbles, Swansea

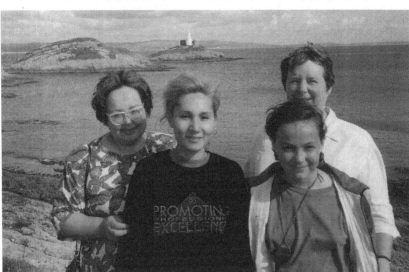

them into England. Goulnara talked of her 'enemies' and the people who were jealous that she had got the job. Getting visas was a nightmare. On two occasions our passports and my visa, which the authorities had confiscated and were holding 'to complete procedures', were mysteriously lost, and only found again on the intervention of the British chargé d'affaires.

During my first trip to Kazakhstan I stayed in a hotel in Alma Ata. I talked with the doorman because he was the only person who spoke a little English. He said he was a paediatrician who worked extra shifts at the hotel because the pay was better than at the hospital! The second time, I stayed at Goulnara's home. This was a tiny flat that she shared with her parents, her younger sister and her daughter. The flat was in a typical Soviet-style block near the centre of the city. On a later visit the team rented an apartment. This apartment was infested with cockroaches, so as we opened the door we switched on the light so they would scurry back into their cracks before we dared enter. Getting around was scary, particularly when alone, as was sometimes required. We were warned not to try to walk anywhere, especially after dark. We were provided with a car and a driver, but getting into a car with a driver who spoke no English in order to travel to a totally unknown destination was pretty frightening.

However, despite the basic facilities and communication challenges the people we met were wonderful. I have never before or since experienced such hospitality. Everywhere we went we were greeted by huge banquets and showered with gifts. They had so little, but whatever they had – sometimes their own most treasured possessions – they wanted to give us. There were just two problems with the banquets. The first was that an empty plate was not allowed, so as soon as you emptied it, it was immediately refilled. To say that you did not want any more was seen as a slur on the hospitality, so we ate until fit to burst. The second was the custom that after every course someone was required to stand up and give a speech followed by a toast – and every toast involved completely emptying the glass of vodka. I pleaded allergy to alcohol, but on more than one occasion we had to carry a very drunk colleague to the car provided to take us home!

On my last visit I was entertained by the Torgabaiev family, whose daughter Anel came to stay at our home in Reading for a few weeks – I remember her reaction when we collected her from Heathrow airport – it was late evening and she was completely bowled over by all the lights. (There was no street lighting or lights in public buildings after dark in Alma Ata.) Anel's father described himself as 'Professor of Re-animatology', which turned out to mean Professor of Intensive Care. During my weekend with them I went down with a terrible cold. I coughed and coughed and my eyes and nose streamed. Professor Torgobaiev made me sit in an armchair and got out what he called his 'magic box'. He proceeded to insert acupuncture needles into my forehead, under my eyes and into my wrists. Within minutes the coughing stopped and my eyes and nose stopped streaming.

Leaving Middlesex University

By the end of 1995 I was completely exhausted and burnt out. Despite Professor Torgabaiev's treatment, I returned from Kazakhstan with a hacking cough and for the first time in years I went 'off sick'. My GP diagnosed asthma caused by the environmental pollution in Alma Ata, and work-related stress. The internal politics and jockeying for position within the University were considerable and it was not a happy time. I had to face challenges by Vice Chancellor David Melville about many issues, but I received great support from Liz Clark, and from RCN General Secretary Christine Hancock, who accompanied me on the many meetings with him. Fortunately, I found an ally in the University's Deputy Vice-Chancellor, Professor Ken Goulding.

In addition to these challenges, the School was about to be restructured, and my two best team members had decided to move on: Kevin to become the first Professor of Psychiatric Nursing at the Institute of Psychiatry, King's College London, and Liz to the RCN to establish its higher education distance learning provision. I shall always be grateful for the support they gave me while they were at Middlesex, and proud of what they went on to achieve.

In 1995 the Queen made me a Dame, my old alma mater University College London made me a Fellow, and Middlesex University gave me a 0% bonus in the new performance-related pay scheme! I had had enough.

The 6 years I had spent at Middlesex were the toughest of my whole career. Luckily for me, in 1996 the University offered voluntary early retirement to many staff members, and I decided to accept. On the day of my departure I went to say goodbye to Ken Goulding, and a few days later he wrote: 'Thank you for coming to see me last week. I much appreciated the fact that you did so, given the way I know you feel about your time at Middlesex. I sincerely hope and believe that, in time, the University overall will recognise what you achieved here to be much more significant than is currently acknowledged. I certainly do already and will miss your advice on issues related to the NHS and to the education of nurses and midwives.' The time did come. Eight years later he wrote to me again, this time to offer me an honorary doctorate. When I expressed surprise, his reply was: 'Call it compensation!'

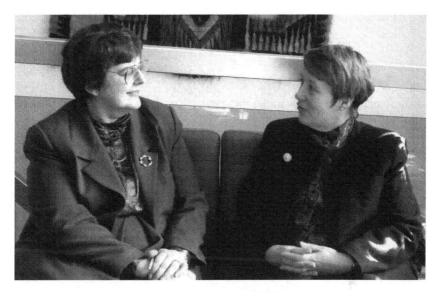

With Norma Lang 1991

CHAPTER 6: A NEW WORLD: NURSING INFORMATICS

As part of my retirement package I negotiated a sabbatical. I wanted to pursue my interest in standardised nursing language. I had begun work on this with Gretta Styles and Norma Lang while working on the ICN's International Classification for Nursing Practice (ICNP) project back in 1990, but had never had the time to properly develop it. I applied for, and won, two scholarships – a Florence Nightingale scholarship to look at clinical information systems and the development of standardised nursing languages in the USA, and a Churchill Fellowship to do the same thing in Europe. This opportunity was to open up whole new world for me. It also introduced me to a new circle of friends and colleagues who became my main reference group for the next 10 years.

I began by attending the biennial conference of the North American Nursing Diagnosis Association (NANDA), held that year in Pittsburgh. It was there that the penny dropped that nursing diagnosis was the key to understanding nursing practice and to identifying nursing outcomes. How on earth did I previously practise without it? I became more involved with

NANDA and with what was happening in the USA, and later became a member of NANDA's Board of Directors. In 2002 I received their Founders Award for promoting these ideas across Europe – an award I feel I never deserved, because in spite of my best efforts UK nurses still do not understand or see the relevance of the concept. As a result of this lack of understanding, in the UK the development of electronic health records still does not include nursing and we are light-years behind the rest of the world in nursing informatics.

The conference helped me to identify the places I wanted to visit and the people I wanted to meet during my sabbatical. I spent a wonderful month at the University of Iowa where Gloria Bulechek, Joanne McCloskey, Connie Delaney, Sue Moorhead, Meridean Mass and Marti Craft-Rosenberg were working on the nursing interventions and nursing outcomes classifications (NIC and NOC). I was privileged to be welcomed as a member of the team, and I learnt a great deal. I saw the clinical information system actually working in the university hospital, and saw the difference it made. What excited me most, however, was the continuous and collaborative involvement of all the academic staff, their clinical associates, and their postgraduate students in the project, and how this work was undertaken in addition to their normal teaching and research activities, often during lunchtimes and at odd times of the day; the continuous intellectual 'stretching' was exhausting but wonderfully stimulating.

I was especially keen to find out more about the leadership provided by the American Nurses Association, which had been working on the issue of standardised languages since the 1970s. This was in sharp contrast with the RCN, which back in 1991 had laughed at the development of the ICNP and shown no interest in nursing informatics, believing informatics to be a role for 'techies' rather than nurses. The American Nurses Association had a specific Steering Committee for Databases Supporting Nursing Practice, chaired by Judith (Judy) Warren. The Committee had developed a system for accrediting nursing languages and getting them into the National Library of Medicine's Unified Medical Language System. This move subsequently enabled nursing concepts to be included in SNOMED-CT, which has since become the global standardised terminology for health and healthcare. Although the RCN may not recognise it, UK nursing owes a great debt to the work of the American Nurses Association in this field. Judy agreed to meet me at the pool of the hotel where we were staying so that she could explain the system to me. The meeting was supposed to last for an hour or so but we talked all day. Some 8 hours later Judy's husband Ed had to drag us in for dinner. We were both sunburned because we were too engrossed to come in out of the sun!

Many of the people I met subsequently came to stay with me in Swansea, where they gave their expertise freely and free of charge in masterclasses and teaching sessions on nursing outcomes and clinical information systems. Despite the fact that the speakers were world leaders in their fields, however, they were totally ignored by nurses in Wales.

After the USA I turned my attention to Europe, where I already had good contacts because the previous year, following the first European Conference on Nursing Diagnosis held in Copenhagen in 1993, we had established a new pan-European organisation called the Association for Common European Nursing Diagnosis Interventions and Outcomes or ACENDIO; Randi Mortensen from Denmark became its first President and I became its first Secretary and subsequently President. Through my involvement in ACENDIO, I visited the Nordic countries, Belgium and the Netherlands.

The MIE96 (Medical Informatics Europe) conference that was held that year in Copenhagen provided a golden opportunity to find out more about what was happening in Denmark, Norway, Sweden, Finland and Iceland. It soon became clear that the US was not the only country making progress in informatics. In Iceland, Asta Thoroddsen was testing the emerging ICNP in a clinical setting; I was privileged a few years later to be the external examiner for her doctoral thesis on the project, and Iceland has now fully implemented a clinical information system that incorporates nursing. In both Sweden and Finland, the national nurses associations were working on projects. In Denmark, in addition to the work of the Danish Institute of Health and Nursing Research (then part of the Danish Nurses' Organisation), the National Board of Health was developing classification systems for both nursing diagnosis and nursing interventions. In Sweden, Margreta Ehnfors and Anna Erenberg were developing a classification system called the VIPS system. In Finland, Anneli Ensio was working with Virginia Saba's Clinical Care Classification (CCC) System. I went to Belgium to talk with Walter Sermeus, the nurse leader of the team that had developed the Belgian Nursing Minimum Data Set that had been used since 1989 to provide data used for funding all Belgian hospitals. I also met Government Chief Nurse Anita Simoens, whose interest and commitment had clearly been influential. In the Netherlands I saw clinical information systems being developed or used in several hospitals, including the university hospitals at Groningen and Leiden, and at Vaught (the oldest psychiatric hospital in the Netherlands), and the paper-based but nevertheless very effective system used by the community nursing service in Breda. I talked with nurses in the Universities of Leuven (Walter Sermeus and George Evers), Groningen, where Theo Dassen was leading a team working on the validation of several nursing diagnoses, and Maastricht, where Harry van der Bruggen and Maike Groen were working on the definition of nursing outcomes. While at Groningen I also visited a nursing home for elderly people with dementia, following up on my interest in older people.

I did not get a lot of sleep, but as I sat on trains and in airports, questions kept bubbling up in my mind. What explains the similarities and differences I have found? What drives development in those countries where there is such a lot going on, but is missing in neighbouring countries where there is nothing? Why is the UK so far behind? In a paper presented to the 1998 NANDA conference held in St Louis, I suggested some possible answers:

- Driving forces: in all countries, the development of computerised information systems for management and financial purposes; in the USA the requirements of the quality assurance and accreditation systems; in Belgium and Switzerland, the development of nationally-mandated minimum data sets; in Sweden, the 1986 Patient Records Act, which requires nurses to record their care alongside that of the physician, and government guidance that identifies diagnosis as part of nursing care.
- The role of the national nurses association in each country: in the USA, the contribution of the American Nurses Association, and in particular the incorporation of nursing diagnosis into the American Nurses Association Standards of Nursing Practice and the work of the Steering Committee for Databases Supporting Nursing Practice, has been enormous. The support of the national nurses associations in Nordic countries has also been very important.
- The way that 'the nursing process' is taught to students and used in practice.
- The system of nursing education.

Part of the reason we are so far behind is that in the UK these factors are weak or missing. There is no legislation about nursing documentation, and such guidance as is provided by the regulatory body – the Nursing and Midwifery Council – is extraordinarily weak. In spite of my efforts, the RCN has offered no leadership on this issue. The nursing process as it is practised (if at all) in the UK is stuck in the 1970s version as a linear four-step process involving assessment, planning, implementation, and evaluation. It does not include diagnosis, goals or outcomes. Standardised nursing language is not used; indeed, it is confused with standardising nursing practice and is therefore positively rejected. In addition to this, nursing education is dominated by employer rather than professional perspectives. The concept of what nursing is – the paradigm that sees nursing as tasks rather than a process of decision-making – underpins all of these reasons.

My intention was to dig a little hole for myself and spend the next few years just indulging my academic interests, and writing a book or two. Once again it was not to be. As part of my retirement 'package' I was allocated a career consultant who tried to recreate me as a 'consultant' – never a realistic hope for someone wedded to public sector values and ideals! While I was in Iowa I received a phone call from her, telling me that there was a Chair in Nursing post being advertised at Swansea University. I was happy where I was, and pointed this out; however, she persisted, pointing out the fact that my family came from Swansea and saying: 'I know you well enough now to know that if some wimp got it and you hadn't applied, you'd be furious.' She was right. 'Tell you what I'll do,' she said, 'I'll send them your CV and explain that you are in the USA. You've nothing to lose – only a first class stamp, and I'll treat you to that. If they're interested they will call you for interview. And that means you get an expenses-paid trip home. If they don't like you, well at least you've had a free trip home. And if they like you they'll offer you the job. And even if they offer you the job, if you don't like it you don't have to accept it!'

The interview was fixed for a Monday morning. The day before I was due to be in Washington for a very important American Nurses Association meeting that I was determined not to miss, so I booked an overnight flight, having explained that I could not get to Swansea in time for a morning interview. The plan was for Roger to collect me at Heathrow, take me home to Reading for a wash and brush up, and then I would catch the train to Swansea to arrive early afternoon. The plane was 3 hours late into Heathrow. Roger was still there, patiently waiting for me, but by this time there was no chance I would catch my train to Wales. 'Well, that's that. You win some and you lose some,' I said. 'Rubbish,' he responded. 'Get in the car. I'm driving you to Swansea.'

We got there in time. I was offered the job, and I accepted.

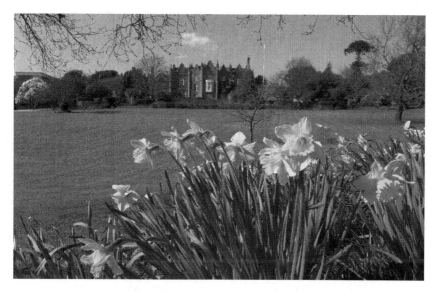

Swansea University in springtime

CHAPTER 7: HIRAETH: HOME TO WALES

I took up my post at Swansea University on 1 January 1997 – the University's first Professor of Nursing. I set out my stall, as new professors in those days were expected to do, in an inaugural public lecture. The title was Florence Nightingale's famous remark 'The elements of nursing are all but unknown'. I began by summarising all I had learnt over the previous decade about the importance of standardised language, based on Norma Lang's much quoted remark: 'If you can't name it, you can't control it, finance it, teach it, research it, or put it into public policy.' I argued the need for more basic research in nursing – identifying and naming its elements. This is the first step of theory development in other disciplines but is not well developed in British nursing research, which seems to be more concerned with nurses, their opinions and roles rather than with nursing, i.e. the conditions that nurses know about and can treat. Then, since the Spice Girls' song 'Wannabe' was number one in the charts, I decided to tell them 'what I want, what I really, really want'. I set out a potential research programme based on identifying a multidisciplinary general practice team whose members would record their diagnoses, interventions and outcomes using the same standardised language in a computerised information system. If the database thus created was then analysed using the data-mining techniques I had seen in operation in the USA, we could identify the different contributions to care made by different members of the team, and in particular identify their outcomes. Within a few months the Welsh Office of Research and Development had taken up the idea and incorporated it into a project called SCIPICT, which it put out to tender. It then awarded the contract to another research team! Despite this, I wanted to pursue the idea of identifying and measuring nursing outcomes through the retrospective analysis of nursing data. To my surprise and horror, I found there were no databases containing nursing data to analyse. The nearest thing available was the Child Health Record System (CHRS) in which health visitors recorded every child's immunisations and developmental reviews. However, the system did not record any information about what the health visitor actually did (the education, support and counselling that are the core of the health visitor's work).

My first PhD student, Marjorie Talbot, took on the task of finding out how this system actually worked and whether it could be used to further our aims. She traced the whole process by first observing health visitors during visits to see what they recorded in the CHRS paper forms and comparing it with what they wrote in their own records. She then worked with the coding clerks who coded and transferred what the health visitors had written from the paper forms into the computer system, and then examined how the data were aggregated, analysed and used. What she found was that the data retained in the CHRS database were not worth the paper they were originally written on: at every step in the process there were errors and omissions, and the health visiting data were gradually excluded, until all that was left was minimal (often inaccurate) medical data. Using the record of one child as a detailed case study, she was able to show that the original records of the health visitor provided evidence of child abuse, which was missed because the relevant data were systematically excluded from the official record.

On my second day at Swansea, a typically cold and rainy January day, I wandered into the University bookshop. The only other customer was a man whom I recognised from previous activities in Wales. It was Rodney Hughes, whom I had known as Chief Nursing Officer for Pembrokeshire. He had taken early retirement from the NHS and won a scholarship to fulfil a long-held ambition to do a PhD. In his early career he had been a clinical nurse specialist in spinal injuries. He believed, and wanted to demonstrate, that in this field of nursing the nurse made a particular contribution independent from that of the doctor or the physiotherapist, but he did not know how to go about it. Over a cup of coffee I persuaded him to use the work on interventions and outcomes that I had seen in Iowa, and he became my second PhD student. As the first phase of his work, he undertook a Delphi study (a structured communication method that relies on a panel of experts) among the senior nurses in all of the special spinal injuries units in the UK, asking them to identify in their own words the patient conditions they treated independently and the interventions they used. The first round identified a consensus on a number of conditions and interventions, expressed in a great variety of terms. He then fed back what they had identified using standardised terms (NANDA nursing diagnoses and Nursing Interventions Classification interventions) and asked whether these terms accurately expressed the concepts the senior nurses had identified. The use of the standardised terms greatly improved the level of consensus. He then returned to work for 6 months as a staff nurse in a spinal injuries unit, observing what the nurses did for what conditions, and how they documented their work. He was able to demonstrate several important findings: first, some of the specific independent contributions made by the nurses (e.g. in bowel and bladder care) and their outcomes; second, the huge amount of psychosocial care that he observed that was not recorded in documentation and therefore was unrecognised; and third, through the use of case studies, that patients who had the same medical diagnosis had very different nursing diagnoses, to which the nurses responded with very different interventions.

The concept of nursing diagnoses that are distinct from medical diagnoses is fundamental to understanding nursing practice, to developing nursing knowledge, and to identifying nursing outcomes. Without it, nursing remains task-oriented or directed by medical diagnoses. Sadly UK nurses are stuck in the outmoded idea that only doctors diagnose. In reality all professions, or indeed anyone who uses a problem-solving process of decision making, diagnose; the only difference is in what they diagnose. Each discipline diagnoses conditions that they 'know about' and can treat – so doctors diagnose and treat diseases, while car mechanics diagnose and treat broken down cars. Nurses diagnose and treat the patient conditions that they know about such as impaired skin integrity, self-care deficits, care-giver role strain, etc. These conditions are defined by the American Nurses Association as 'human responses to actual or potential threats to health', a definition that is incorporated into the definition of nursing in many countries. While nursing diagnosis is used in most countries, UK nurses do not understand or use the concept. I was therefore initially thrilled when I found district nurses in Newport using a documentation system (called Compass) in which the front page had a space for writing in the nursing diagnosis. Since the data contained in the nurses' paper records were transferred into a computerised database, here was the database for which I had been searching. I asked for a printout of the ten most common diagnoses. My joy was short-lived. The most commonly listed included 'cancer' (a medical diagnosis), 'dressing' (a nursing intervention), and something called 'venous puncture' that I misread as 'venepuncture' (a common nursing procedure). It was not until later that we discovered that the coding clerks (whose job was simply to convert the nurses' words to numerical codes using a codebook) were allocating the nursing term 'venepuncture' to the code for 'venous puncture', which is a rather rare type of injury to a vein. I still smile as I imagine some poor epidemiologist trying to work out why there is such a high incidence of this rare phenomenon in south east Wales!

Since I could find no ready-made nursing databases to analyse, I decided I would have to create one to use as a test-bed. At about this time, health visitors in Swansea were becoming increasingly worried about their documentation and a study day had been organised to improve their skills. I went too, and was horrified by what I learnt. The whole day was taken up with sessions led by a lawyer about the documentation required for child protection; there was no consideration of the role of documentation for professional purposes. The greatest embarrassment was that the lawyer, who was unaware of my presence, was recommending the approach that I had developed in Berkshire 15 years previously – but had got it all wrong! The positive outcome was that I identified a group of health visitors who were prepared to work with me to develop and test a system of documentation for health visiting that would properly reflect their work and enable them to identify and measure outcomes.

One of these health visitors was Jean Christensen, who became the project leader and a good friend. We decided to try the Omaha System originally developed by Karen Martin for the Visiting Nurses Association of Omaha during the 1970s. Karen was already a member of my USA 'informatics reference group'; I had met her several times at conferences and she visited us in Swansea, so we had ready access to advice. Over the next 4 years we tested the system, modified and validated the terminology for UK use, and were able to demonstrate for the very first time that health visitors did actually make a difference in terms of changes in their clients' knowledge and behaviour. We tested our system by using it to evaluate the Swansea Sure Start programme, a programme of intensive health visiting for selected vulnerable families. In the final phase of the project, supported for the first time by a Welsh Assembly Government grant, we developed a prototype to be used on a laptop.

I believed, and I still believe, that we had developed a useful tool. We published and presented our work at conferences, locally, nationally and internationally but no one in NHS Wales was interested. Jean, by now the most knowledgeable nurse informaticist in Wales, went back to work as a field-level health visitor. With great determination, but little support from her employer, she later completed her PhD. Ten years on we still have no data about what health visitors do or what they achieve.

I really enjoyed the opportunity to teach, especially to work with people who really wanted to learn. A group of health visitors in Ammanford wanted to find out whether introducing pre-natal visits would improve the incidence and length of breastfeeding, and they wanted to learn how to do a randomised clinical trial. We therefore set up a trial using as the intervention a pre-natal visit with a specially designed teaching pack. It fell apart when, in typical Welsh village fashion, mothers in the control group (who were not getting the extra visit and the teaching pack) found out that their friends were getting something special and borrowed their teaching pack to read, just to be sure that they were not missing out. This provided an excellent lesson about the difficulties of doing randomised controlled trials, especially in nursing. It was also an opportunity to demonstrate the value of retrospective analysis of nursing records as an alternative method.

I undertook several projects commissioned by the Welsh Assembly Government, but it was not a good experience. For example, with a large project team I worked on a review of health visiting and school health services in Wales. What we found in Wales in 2000 was very different from what I had found in my MPhil study in Berkshire in the 1970s. It was also very different from the services I had been responsible for in England. In Wales over the previous decade (or perhaps longer) health visiting and school nursing had been sorely neglected and had almost withered away. Services varied widely across Wales. Neither health authorities nor trusts could tell us exactly what services were currently being delivered, to whom, or by whom; moreover, they had no way of finding out because their information systems were so inadequate. Three years earlier the Audit Commission had recommended that the Department of Health and the Welsh Office should 'provide renewed leadership in developing a framework for measuring activity and outcomes in community health services'. We found that little progress had been made in implementing this recommendation, and we in our turn recommended that 'the Assembly should give urgent consideration to the development on an all-Wales basis of appropriate clinical information systems for community health services'. Fifteen years later this has still not been achieved.

We identified a lack of professional leadership and strategic direction; only half of the trusts had a health visitor at a senior level with strategic responsibility for the service, and in three trusts the most senior health visitor was a field-level practitioner. We found that there was no specification of what services should be offered, and neither the health authorities nor the health visitors themselves were clear about the meaning of 'public health' or the health visitors' role in it. We concluded that although the health visiting and school health services had the potential to deliver the Assembly's agenda for health in Wales, they were 'underdeveloped, undermanaged, and under resourced'. The report was quietly shelved.

A more successful commission was the work on fundamentals of care. In England in 2001, the Department of Health had produced a document entitled *Essence of Care*, which was designed to tackle concerns being expressed about standards of basic nursing care. It identified nine areas of care, and provided a benchmarking toolkit that would enable nurses to identify best practice and compare their own standards with other places. In Wales a decision was made to 'dragonise' the English document under the title *Fundamentals of Care*. A working party was established and I won the tender to write the document. Before this, however, various changes had already been decided: the benchmarking approach was rejected, one of the areas of concern (record keeping) had been dropped and other areas added. There was little I could do to change the content areas, but I did persuade the working party to use the approach to standards development that I had used in Berkshire some 20 years earlier. On the Friday afternoon after the text had finally been agreed ready for the printer, I received a phone call to say that the word 'standard' could no longer be used because it was being used to mean something different in the document about minimum standards of care in social services which had just been published. This meant *Fundamentals of Care* had to be completely re-written using different terminology. The first edition was launched in 2003 and 11 years later *Fundamentals of Care* was still used throughout Wales as the framework for standards of nursing care; I did not know whether to be flattered or horrified that after all the changes of the past decade, it was still being used in its original form. Only now, in 2015, is being reviewed and revised.

Towards undergraduate nursing education in Wales

Devolution in 1999 resulted in a flurry of documents and strategies in all four countries of the UK, especially in health and education, which were the main newly-devolved responsibilities. Gradually differences emerged. I became involved in several of the committees and taskforces that were established on primary care, informatics, services for older people, and nursing. In Wales, work on a strategy for nursing had begun before devolution, led by the Chief Nursing Officer for Wales, Marion Bull, who was about to retire. *Realising the Potential: A Strategic Framework for Nursing Midwifery and Health Visiting in Wales into the 21st Century* was scheduled for publication early in 1999, but was delayed by the new requirement for translation into Welsh. At the last minute, another barrier was introduced: the new political protocol required that the Wales document could not be published before the equivalent England document, which had not yet been written. Donna Mead, who had led the editorial team, and I happened to be attending a reception in London as part of the ICN centennial conference when the message came through. Donna immediately left the reception to return to Wales to argue the case with Jane Hutt, the new Welsh Minister of Health, and Rosemary Kennedy, the incoming Chief Nursing Officer. The result was that a document for England (*Making a Difference: Strengthening the Nursing, Midwifery and Health Visiting Contribution to Health and Health Care*) was hurriedly written, and the document for Wales was published a few days later. Despite the delays, *Realising the Potential* was in fact the very first document published by the newly-formed National Assembly for Wales.

Realising the Potential has provided a vision of nursing and a strategic framework for the development of nursing in Wales for more than a decade. I believe that its success has been due in great measure to the fact that, unlike the English document, it was developed in consultation with the profession in Wales – more than 5000 nurses, midwives and health visitors took part in the consultation – as well as members of the public and organisations representing the professions and the NHS. The strategic goal, which became almost a mantra, was: 'To realise the full potential of nursing, midwifery and health visiting in order to meet in collaboration with others the future health needs of people in Wales.'

The initial document was followed by a series of Briefing Papers on selected areas of nursing. The most important one was *Creating the potential: A Plan for Education*, which set out the strategy for nursing education. *Realising the Potential* had already coined the term 'graduateness' to describe the cognitive skills that would be required by the nurse of the future, and had explicitly stated: 'This means an all graduate entry to nursing and midwifery.' This was, and continues to be, a controversial proposal. I have always been in favour of graduate entry to nursing, and have written extensively and spoken at many conferences in support of it. I have always argued that, contrary to popular belief, it has much less to do with enhancing the status of nursing than, as *Realising the Potential* argues, with the level of cognitive skills in critical thinking and clinical decision-making that nursing practice in the 21st century requires. I do not believe that the decisions required in nursing are less complex than those required in physiotherapy or occupational therapy (which have had graduate entry for many years) or even medicine. There is no evidence whatsoever that cognitive skills are incompatible with care and compassion, or with a reluctance to undertake the so-called 'basic' nursing care, such as feeding or washing patients. There is no evidence that graduate nurses are 'too posh to wash' or 'too clever to care', but there is an increasing body of evidence that better educated nurses achieve better outcomes for patients.

Wales achieved the Creating the Potential target of all pre-registration nursing education to be at undergraduate level by 2004, and now has 10 years of evidence that it works. England is a decade behind, with undergraduate level preparation becoming mandatory only from September 2013.

In an article in the *Nursing Standard* of 1 September 1999, I challenged two of the basic assumptions of *Making a Difference*. The first was the complaint that 'newly qualified nurses and midwives are coming onto the wards without the full range of skills required for effective practice'. I argued that the idea that initial preparation should produce at the moment of registration a practitioner who has the full range of skills across any setting is unrealistic. We do not expect it of doctors or teachers or any other professionals, all of whom require a period of consolidation after initial registration. What we do need at the point of registration is practitioners who are safe, know their limits, and can adapt quickly to circumstances; research shows that within 6 months of qualification graduate nurses' technical skills are at least as good as nurses who have been trained by the old method to undertake tasks, and they are better able to take responsibility and to make decisions. I also challenged the assumption that the purpose of pre-registration preparation is to meet the immediate needs of NHS hospital wards, rather than providing the knowledge, skills and attitudes that will enable nurses to respond to people's health needs wherever they present themselves, whatever the organisational setting, throughout a career that may last 40 years.

I pointed to what I consider to be a sinister aspect of the *Making a Difference* proposals – the statement that 'we want to strengthen the links between education and NHS employment [...] to deliver a nurse training system that is more responsive to the needs of the NHS'. Who, I asked, is 'we'? I saw this as a blatant expression of government control of what I believe should be a professional responsibility. And why only the needs of the NHS, when a third of all nurses work outside the NHS, for example in care homes for frail older people, whose numbers are increasing while the number of NHS beds is falling? Over the past decade the validity of these concerns has been confirmed. Nursing education, however, is still a contested issue.

Meanwhile, in December 1997 my interest in the care of older people was kicked into action again by my appointment to the Royal Commission on Long Term Care. At first I was not too pleased, because the terms of reference focussed on funding whereas I was more interested in care, but a royal warrant is an invitation not to be ignored. My anxiety was dispelled at our first meeting when our chairman, Sir Stewart (now Lord) Sutherland, from his background as a moral philosopher, set out the principles to which we were to work: to create a fair, just and transparent system for funding and delivering long-term care. The 12 commissioners included two nurses, myself and Claire Rayner – better known as an author and popular agony aunt – and two other women, Iona Heath, a London GP, and Mary Marshall, then Head of the Dementia Services Development Centre at Stirling University. The others were very distinguished men drawn from the fields of the law, business and public service. The economics journalist David Lipsey was also a commissioner. Over time we came to recognise David as a 'mole'. From the early stages of our work he was hell-bent on destroying it. In her autobiography *How Did I Get Here From There?*, Claire Rayner describes our anger when we discovered what was happening. David went on to write the 'Note of Dissent' that enabled the government to reject our recommendations, and has campaigned against them ever since. What made me most angry was that in the first Honours List after our report was published, it was he and the one other commissioner whom he persuaded to sign the Note of Dissent, Joel Joffe, who were rewarded with seats in the House of Lords.

The Royal Commission report was entitled *With Respect to Old Age: Long Term Care – Rights and Responsibilities*. Its main recommendation was to separate the costs of living (board and lodging) from the costs of care: 'the costs of care for those individuals who need it should be split between living costs, housing costs, and personal care. Personal care should be available after an assessment, according to need and paid for from general taxation: the rest should be subject to a co-payment according to means.' The media, fed by the dissenting commissioners and the government spin-doctors, misrepresented this as 'free care for all'. In fact, we defined personal care (a term we chose only to avoid the confusion over 'health' and 'social' care) very carefully as:

'...care that directly involves touching a person's body (and therefore incorporates issues of intimacy, personal dignity and confidentiality) and is distinct both from treatment/therapy (a procedure a procedure deliberately intended to cure or ameliorate a pathological condition) and from indirect care such as home help or the provision of meals. [...] Personal care would cover all direct care related to:

- *Personal toilet (washing, bathing, skin care, personal presentation, dressing and undressing and skin care);*
- *Eating and drinking (as opposed to obtaining and preparing food and drink);*
- *Managing urinary and bowel functions (including maintaining continence and managing incontinence);*
- *Managing problems associated with immobility;*
- *Management of prescribed treatment (e.g. administration and monitoring medication);*
- *Behaviour management and ensuring personal safety (for example those with cognitive impairment – minimising stress and risk).*

Personal care also includes the associated teaching, enabling, psychological support from a knowledgeable and skilled professional and assistance with cognitive functions (e.g. reminding, for those with dementia) that are needed either to enable a person to do these things for himself/herself or to enable a relative to do them for him/her.'

This section of the Commission's Report drew heavily on a paper that I had submitted on the nature of nursing, and it included the specific statement that: 'It [the Commission's definition of personal care] falls within the internationally recognised definition of nursing.' I was referring to Virginia Henderson's definition of the unique function of the nurse as: 'to assist the individual, sick or well, in the performance of those activities contributing to health or its recovery or to peaceful death, that he would perform unaided if he had the necessary strength, will, or knowledge. And to do this in such a way as to help him gain independence as rapidly as possible.'

I have always argued, and continue to argue, that personal care is nursing care, although it may be delivered by people who are not nurses. Its knowledge base, which is required for the assessment of nursing need and the prescription of nursing care, is nursing knowledge. It is a travesty that in our present system personal care is prescribed (commissioned) by social workers who do not have this knowledge because their training and knowledge base are quite different.

Over 15 years and numerous reports later, I believe that none has identified a better solution than ours. Scotland, under the wise leadership of Sir Stewart, has implemented our recommendation. This has not been without difficulties, but it shows what can be done, even in times of austerity.

International work

During my time at Swansea University I continued to maintain my international contacts. I visited Malta to advise the Government on the development of community nursing. In the University of Mahidol in Bangkok, I planned and delivered a module on leadership in their new doctoral programme for nurses. Work on the ICN's ICNP continued, with workshops in Mexico and Taiwan, and with groups in Japan and Sweden, in addition to meetings at the ICN headquarters in Geneva. In 2006 I was asked by the University of Primorska in Slovenia to help in the development of a new Masters programme for nurses; for the next 5 years I visited every year to deliver a core module on evidence-based practice.

Japan

In 2002 I went to Japan to work with the Japanese Nursing Association on the ICN's International Classification for Nursing Project but, as always, used the opportunity to learn what I could about other things. My hostess, Shigemi Kamatsuri, was eager to show me all things Japanese. One weekend we went to Kyoto, where we stayed in a traditional Japanese guest-house called a ryokan. It was quite an experience. Our room was like the one in the Bond film *You Only Live Twice*, with sliding walls (fusuma) and tatami flooring. There were no beds, only two futons on a shelf to be laid on the floor at bedtime, plus a dressing gown (yukata) and cotton slippers that we were expected to wear all the time. Food was served in the room on a table that emerged from the floor to a height of about a foot. I cannot say that I enjoyed Japanese food, especially the green tea that was served at every meeting, and getting down to floor level to eat was a major challenge. The toilet included a heated seat that could be raised for an elderly user, and several buttons for extra facilities I did not dare to explore. I was, however, grateful that the toilet was not one of the traditional sort – a hole in the floor over which you had to squat. Shigemi told me that hip problems among older people were an increasing issue in Japan. This was thought to be associated with the increased use of Western-style toilets that avoid the need for squatting.

I had the opportunity to discuss with local staff the system for funding and providing care for older people in Japan, and I visited a care home. I believe the UK could learn some lessons from Japan when it comes to the provision of such services. Access to a variety of community-based services, including residential and nursing care, is available to all those over the age of 65 years on the basis of need alone, as assessed by a standardised nationwide assessment tool; income and wealth are not taken into consideration in the assessment, which is undertaken by nurses. Funding comes from a system of compulsory social insurance, but the clever trick is that contributions begin at the age of 40 years, when most people can see immediate benefit for their parents or someone they know. Those who use services are also required to make co-payments of up to 10% of the costs of care. At the care home I was at first horrified to see the huge communal bathroom; however, I changed my mind when back at the hotel I was treated to the traditional Japanese experience of a bath, which – rather like I imagine the Roman bathing experience to have been – was a communal and social experience that occurred only after an initial body cleansing procedure had been carefully completed. From this I learnt the lesson never to make assumptions based on one's own cultural stereotypes.

I also had the opportunity to shadow a health visitor for a home visit to a family with a toddler and a new baby. The living room had no furniture other than a shelf around the four walls on which were stacked the TV and other family possessions and, in the middle of the room, what appeared to be a large table about a foot high covered with a heavy tablecloth. I watched while the mother undressed the baby and the health visitor examined him, just as I would have done as a health visitor in the UK. The mother dressed the baby again, wrapped him in a shawl, and then put him under the table! The mystery was solved when we were invited to sit down with our legs under the table to take the ubiquitous green tea: under the 'table', which is called a kotatsu, was an electric heater, which constituted the house's central heating system.

Towards retirement

The only downside of my time at the School of Health Sciences was the Head of School, Barbara Green. At times she was the nicest and kindest person you could imagine. At other times she would take a dislike to someone (in particular, but not exclusively, to me) and would behave quite viciously towards that person. I learned to treat it as water off a duck's back, but I know that it embarrassed my colleagues. Perhaps she saw me as a threat in spite of my explanation that having once suffered (at Middlesex) the challenges of the 'faculty dean' role, I had no wish to usurp her or undermine her position. The crunch point was her veto – made quite publicly and explicitly in the statement that it would not happen so long as she was Head of School – on all my efforts to develop a professorial nursing unit like the one I had had at Middlesex University. By the end of 2002 I knew I had achieved all I could in this position and it was time to retire.

I set the date for my retirement as September 2003 to coincide with Roger's planned retirement date. I announced my intention at the ACENDIO conference held earlier that year in Berlin. Most of my 'informatics reference group' colleagues from the USA and all around Europe were there. One said, 'Ooh, can we have a party? And can we all come?' We joked about it, but the idea took root in my head. Somebody said 'It's a helluva long way to come for a party. Is there a conference we can come to? Then I can get somebody to pay my fare!' So the idea of a conference, to be followed by a party, was born.

Nico Oud, who owned a commercial conference-organising business as well as being an ACENDIO member and organiser of the previous ACENDIO conferences, agreed to organise the meeting. I decided that this would be a wonderful opportunity to present to nurses in the UK, especially in Wales, all the expertise from which I had benefited over the past decade. I assembled a stellar cast – from the USA, Sweden, Netherlands, Belgium, Denmark, Finland, Switzerland, Ireland, and the UK. All the speakers – my friends – agreed to work free of charge and to pay their own expenses. And, obviously, they planned to come to the party afterwards! I gave them all the same brief: to describe the development of standardised nursing language and electronic patient records in their own country and to say something about their own personal contribution to it. I asked the retiring Vice Chancellor, who had appointed me and was due to retire on the same day as me, to open the conference and the new Vice Chancellor to close it. I would chair the event.

One of the features of ACENDIO conferences at that time was publication of the full conference proceedings in the form of a book. As the publisher did not have distribution facilities, the books were made available to participants at the time of the conference; this meant that papers had to be presented and the book edited well in advance of the conference. All of the speakers obliged, and within a few months I had edited the book. When I looked at it, I realised that it was a treasure – the only book that described the development of standardised language in so many countries, and in an easily readable form that would be accessible to the average UK nurse reader.

Meanwhile, in spite of extensive marketing efforts, registrations were very slow coming in. Although the conference was targeted at UK, and especially Welsh, nurses, we had registrations from all over the world – except the UK. We offered reduced, and then free, registrations to Welsh nurses. For some reason Barbara Green not only decided not to come herself, but also refused to allow time for any of the School of Health Science staff to come.

The day came when Nico suggested that the conference was not going to cover its costs and should be cancelled. I persuaded him to delay the decision until the very latest date possible, on the promise that if necessary I personally would underwrite it. In particular, I was not prepared to drop the book I had edited so I took a deep breath and transferred the contract with the publisher – a commitment of 20 000 Swiss francs – from Nico's company to me. Fortunately we did not have to cancel the conference, and sales of the book, called *Naming Nursing: Proceedings of the First ACENDIO Ireland/ UK Conference held September 2003 in Swansea, Wales*, recovered almost all of the cost of publication. It is still the only book of its kind.

On the Saturday after the conference finished we held the party. Our house might have been built for parties: it has an open plan ground floor with the living room opening onto a large patio, which in turn gives access to an unused lane, so there was lots of space. The weather was kind. We had a barbecue, a jazz band and a disco. At the conference I had issued an open invitation, so lots of people turned up in addition to those originally invited. A good time was had by all, and even today old friends and colleagues still remind me of it. It was my way of 'going out with a bang'. On 30 September 2003 I retired from my post at Swansea University and Roger retired from his post at Reading University.

PART 3: THE ROYAL COLLEGE OF NURSING: A LIFELONG LOVE AFFAIR

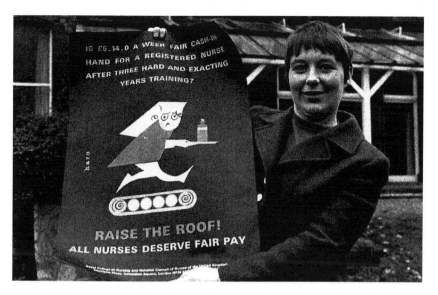

Raise the Roof campaign 1969

CHAPTER 8: BECOMING AN ACTIVIST

At the dinner held to mark the end of my term as President of the Royal College of Nursing (RCN) in October 1994, Richard Bernhard, then the RCN's Head of Legal Services, arranged a *This is Your Life* presentation modelled on the popular TV show in which a celebrity is brought to the studio under some pretext and there confronted with old friends and colleagues who talk about their memories and experiences of him or her. Various dinner guests stood and said their piece, and then Roger was called upon. 'I have been married to June,' he said, 'for 28 years. The trouble is that for 30 years June has been married to the RCN!' It was true. For more than 40 years the RCN was a huge part of my life. I did not plan it that way, but I suppose that having got hooked, I could not let go.

When I moved to Reading in preparation for starting my health visitor training, I started going to meetings of the local RCN branch. Initially I went because I knew I was going to be living in Reading, I was going to be a health visitor in the area, and so it was important to me to develop professional and social contacts. In those days the local matron, who was the Branch President, chaired the meetings, which were quite well attended by all grades of nurse. I was just a staff nurse, and I sat in the back row and said nothing. Nobody knew of my previous activities in the Student Nurses Association and the RCN... until one meeting when the RCN Western Area organiser, Monica Baly, came as guest speaker. I already knew her from my previous activities and she had been one of those who had encouraged me. She saw me in the back row, stopped mid sentence, and said loudly: 'June Hickery, what are you doing here?' And that was it. My cover was blown. She went on to become my good friend and mentor, and I went on to become very involved in the Reading branch as Branch Secretary, Branch Public Relations Officer, Branch Chairman, and Branch Representative at meetings of the RCN Representative Body (RRB).

The 1960s saw big changes in the RCN. Membership was broadened to include male nurses, enrolled nurses and students, and the merger with the National Council of Nurses opened the door to the International Council of Nurses (ICN). The inclusion of male nurses was important for me because it brought me into close contact with some of the greatest leaders the RCN had ever had, and who became my friends and mentors, in particular Trevor Clay, Bob Tiffany, James Smith, Richard Wells and David Rye. By the time the Student Nurses Association was brought into the RCN (1968) there was a new generation of student leaders, but it was the work of my generation that had laid the foundations. Internal reorganisation led to new constitutions for branches and the specialist Sections, which were later to become the Forums. As a health visitor I joined the Public Health Section and the Research Discussion Group (which later became the Research Society), which provided almost all of the support and supervision for my future research career. Under the strong leadership of General Secretary Catherine Hall, Headquarters staff expanded to support the broadened range of activities.

One significant development was the appointment in 1963 of Colonel Douglas de Cent as head of a new Press and Public Relations Department. This led to a sea change in the RCN's relationships with the external world, and in communication with members. While his department had only three members of staff, Colonel de Cent set up a national network of Branch Public Relations Officers, which kept us in touch with developments. This was long before the advent of computers and social media. I was already publishing widely in the nursing press, but soon found myself being interviewed by press and radio and appearing on television as well. One memorable moment was the Michael Parkinson show in which Michael Parkinson 'came out' as having had a vasectomy. Throughout the 70s and the 80s I was often called upon to comment on issues in primary health care and family planning.

All these developments provided the infrastructure for my work in the RCN during the 70s and 80s, but probably the most significant was the replacement of the old Branches Standing Committee by the RRB, the first meeting of which was held in November 1967. I was there as the representative of the Reading Branch, and I participated actively in every single meeting until 2009, including serving as Chair for 4 years (1979–82). Later the RRB changed its name to Congress, which now includes all the surrounding activities as well as the meeting of the Representative Body itself.

The first RCN activity in which I was completely involved was the pay campaign of 1969. The RCN had been involved in campaigning for improvements in nurses' pay and conditions from its very beginning, and had run an organised campaign in 1962, but the response to the report of the Prices and Incomes Board in 1968 led to a much bigger nationwide campaign under the slogan 'Raise the Roof: all nurses deserve fair pay'. The campaign had the benefit of the professional skills of the new Public Relations Department. A ten-point plan of action was carefully prepared. An account of the campaign is included in the book *A Voice for Nurses: A History of the Royal College of Nursing 1916–90:*

The RCN planned a three-stage campaign. The first stage concentrated on national publicity and marshalling the profession's support; the second on regional protest meetings to push the Whitley Council towards a favourable settlement; the third was political, with public pressure on MPs and private negotiations with government officials. Local branches of the RCN received their battle orders and set up action committees. A million copies of a letter stating the nurses' case were circulated for distribution to the public, to be signed and posted to Richard Crossman, the new Secretary of State, Many newspapers co-operated by printing the letter for their readers to cut out.

Professionally-designed campaign posters were prepared with slogans such as 'We stopped putting small boys up chimneys long ago: When do we stop exploiting student nurses?' and 'Job: Chief Nursing Officer. Budget: Millions. Patients: Thousands. Staff: Hundreds. Pay: Peanuts'. Regional meetings were packed out: 3000 in Edinburgh, 6000 in Manchester, and 1500 in Cardiff. Each meeting was accompanied by demonstrations and marches and received wide media coverage. The RRB 1969, held in Harrogate in November, was electric.

Monica Baly was responsible for activities in the Western Region and for organising a mass lobby of MPs. I worked closely with her, helping with the meetings and the marches, taking my 6-month-old son, Andrew, with me. The campaigning worked. We got a pay increase of 20% plus the right to present a further claim the following year.

In 1969 I was elected to Council as representative for the Western Region. I had not expected to be elected so soon, but since I had by now decided that I wanted to be involved, I thought it sensible to get myself known by standing for election. With only one short break I served on the RCN Council for 24 years, first as Regional Representative, then as Chair of Congress, then Deputy President, then President.

I was certainly something different from the usual Council member. I was the youngest and most junior there had ever been. While the other Council members were wearing hats and gloves, I wore trousers. Most revolutionary of all, I was accompanied by a breastfed baby (Gillian was born in January 1972) until I was taken aside by the Chair of Council and asked to make arrangements for her to be minded elsewhere while Council was in session. I remember being so embarrassed that my let-down reflex started, producing a great wet stain on the front of my blouse.

The 1970s

While the most significant issue of the 1970s for the NHS was its reorganisation in 1974, and the most significant issue for nursing was probably the publication in 1972 of the Briggs Report, the issues that dominated my first decade on Council were industrial relations legislation, another pay campaign and internal reorganisation of the RCN.

Reorganisation of the NHS

Although very traumatic for nurses working in the NHS, the reorganisation of the NHS in 1974 provided a great opportunity for me because I was appointed as nurse member of the Berkshire Area Health Authority, a position I retained for almost 10 years. This, alongside my membership of RCN Council, meant that throughout the 70s I was deeply involved in health politics at all levels. By virtue of my RCN and area health authority positions I was appointed to many national committees and taskforces, especially those concerned with primary health care. I spoke at numerous conferences and published several books and numerous articles. I met many wonderful people and learned a great deal that was to stand me in good stead later.

The Briggs Report

In 1970, largely as a result of pressure from the RCN, Secretary of State for Social Services, Richard Crossman, set up a committee under the chairmanship of Professor Asa Briggs 'to review the role of the nurse and the midwife in the hospital and the community and the education and training required for that role, so that the best use is made of available manpower to meet present needs and the needs of an integrated health service'. Christine Hancock, later to become RCN General Secretary, was one of the Committee's two research assistants. The various parts of the RCN were mobilised to prepare evidence and, when the Committee reported in 1972, to comment on the recommendations.

While the Briggs Report was generally welcomed, some of its recommendations were contentious. In particular the 'minority groups' of midwives, health visitors and district nurses felt that their specialist interests were insufficiently protected. By 1979, after 7 years of divisive debate, it became clear that if the profession did not settle its internal differences before the imminent general election, the whole Nurses Midwives and Health Visitors Bill would be lost. At the very last minute the RCN, in the person of David Rye, acted as mediator to persuade the warring parties not to oppose the final reading scheduled for the very next day, which would be the last day of government business before the general election. Although I was very concerned about the future of health visiting, I argued that we should accept what the Bill proposed and should 'sort out the details later'. Elaine Wilkie, Chief Officer of the Council for the Education and Training of Health Visitors, argued strongly for the continuation of the Council, believing that the absorption of health visiting into nursing in the way the Bill proposed would lead to its disempowerment and eventual demise. Although the Bill provided for a special committee for health visiting, with hindsight I was wrong and Elaine Wilkie was right: subsequent developments such as the creation of a part of the register for 'community public health practitioners' led to the loss of the title of 'health visitor', and with it much of the distinct identity of health visiting.

One other sentence in the Briggs Report was highly significant both for the profession and for me in particular. It was that 'nursing should become a research based profession'. This single sentence is often credited with kick-starting the development of nursing research in the 1980s. In particular, it was the trigger for my appointment as Senior Nurse (Research) with the task of improving research awareness among nurses in West Berkshire.

121

Registration as a trade union

Meanwhile, the Industrial Relations Bill introduced by the Heath Government in 1970 exposed the ambiguity of the RCN's role as both a trade union and a professional association. A similar situation was to arise 40 years later as a result of changes in the legislation governing charities. The 1970 Bill required trade unions to register to obtain legal recognition and the right to be recognised by employers for negotiation purposes. The RCN did not want to register as a trade union, but recognised that if it did not register, it would be excluded from one of its most important functions, and it feared a mass exodus of members to unions that did register. If it did register, however, it would lose the considerable financial benefits of its charitable status and would endanger its royal charter. There were heated discussions in RCN Council, but it was the supremely skilled behind-the-scenes political negotiations of General Secretary Catherine Hall and Director of Labour Relations Betty Newstead with the Secretaries of State for Employment (Robert Carr) and Social Services (Sir Keith Joseph) that secured a government amendment to set up a special register for professional associations recognising them as workers' organisations under the Act, with the legal rights and obligations of a trade union, but enabling them to retain their charitable status.

The special register was fiercely opposed by labour members of parliament led by Barbara Castle, who was soon to be in the hot-seat herself, and by the Trades Union Congress (TUC), which urged unions to boycott the Act by refusing to register. The Confederation of Health Service Employees, which registered because it feared that otherwise it would lose members to the RCN, was ejected from the TUC; the TUC did not regard the RCN as a proper union, and holds the same opinion to this day. While the general industrial relations scene was hotting up with a wave of official and unofficial strikes, the 3-day week and pay claims – all culminating in the 'winter of discontent' of 1978/9 – the creation of the special register started a period of open warfare in which the TUC-affiliated unions refused to sit down with the RCN in joint consultative committees at hospital and national level. In some places the animosity amounted to personal threats and even physical violence. In 1974, under the incoming Labour government, the 1971 Act was repealed and replaced by a new Trade Union and Labour Relations Act in which the 'special register' was retained. The RCN finally registered as a trade union, using the special register, in 1977.

The steward scheme

One of the positive consequences for the RCN was that, because the Act required registered organisations to provide representatives in the workplace, it set up a scheme to train and appoint stewards. Following a pilot in the Western Region, a nationwide intensive training scheme was established, and by 1976 there were over 1000 trained stewards elected by their colleagues in each workplace.

One of the first stewards was my dear friend Dora Frost, who was already established as a Congress stalwart. My fondest memory of Dora is the debate in the RRB about district nurses' cars. The government was making it a requirement that district nurses should provide their own cars, and that loans to buy a car should require that the car was totally made in Britain. Dora had members rolling in the aisles with her comparisons with the postal services' little red vans and her images of delivering commodes by Rolls Royce (which was the only car that qualified). I was chairing the meeting but there was absolutely no way I could get her to stop when she exceeded the time allowed to speakers as the audience would have lynched me! Dora was one of the most committed activists the RCN ever had, a charismatic leader, a Council member for 10 years, and later Deputy President of the RCN. She was never afraid to speak out for nurses and nursing, even when it cost her dear: when as a ward sister she spoke out at the RRB about the effect on patient care of the habit of putting in extra beds when the ward was full, she returned home to find that her hoped-for promotion had been vetoed by angry consultants and she had to resign.

The steward scheme was a dramatic success, and it changed the RCN forever. I was disappointed that I was not able to become a steward because at this time I was not working in the NHS except for the occasional shift on the nurse bank, and by the time I was back in the NHS it was at too senior a level to be eligible. I did, however, work hard in Council to secure stewards a position in the RCN structure through the establishment of a National Stewards Committee and its inclusion as an entity in the RRB.

The size and urgency of the task of developing stewards, as required by the Act, meant that everything had to be invested in their development. There was nothing left over for developing other activists, such as the former 'key members' who were mainly involved in developing the 'professional' role of the College. As a result, the stewards – who tended to be more junior in the nursing hierarchy and trade union-focused – swept the board during the next Council elections. To this day experience as a steward is practically a requirement for any office in the RCN. While this was welcome in bringing

Council nearer to the 'ordinary members', a dysfunctional consequence was a lack of experience of strategic planning and financial management among Council members. It is now rare, for example, for Council to include a Director of Nursing among its members.

Internal changes

There were other internal changes. Until then the RCN's top management team had consisted of a triumvirate of the General Secretary, the Labour Relations Secretary, and the Director of Education. The three had operated as a team of equals, all reporting directly to Council. The previous Director of Education, Mary Carpenter, had long argued for greater autonomy for the Education Division to reflect the centrality of the RCN's education function. After her retirement in 1968, all the educational work of the College was brought together into a new Institute of Advanced Nursing Education with Jean McFarlane as its first Director. However, the management consultants brought in to look at the staffing structure recommended that the heads of Education and Labour Relations should report to the General Secretary and Council agreed. Jean refused to accept this loss of autonomy and she resigned – to be immediately snapped up by Professor Alwyn Smith, who was trying to establish nursing at Manchester University. I argued in Council that although this meant that never again would the post of Director of Education of the RCN be the top post in nursing education in the UK, this was exactly right for the nursing profession: the proper place for nursing education was the universities. The rest of the Council were horrified, but I knew that I was right on both counts.

The NHS in crisis: 1973

By 1973 the gains of the 'Raise the Roof' campaign were lost in a period of rampant inflation, the 3-day working week, and the incoming Labour government in which the Secretary of State for Health and Social Services was Barbara Castle. We were exasperated by the slow progress on the implementation of the Briggs Report, and there was deep concern about deteriorating standards of care. We said, not for the first or last time, that the NHS was in crisis.

Nobody who was there will ever forget the 1974 RRB held in Blackpool. On the first night the RRB party was served chicken that proved to be inadequately cooked; by Tuesday half of the participants were suffering from food poisoning. We all had to submit stool specimens to the local public health department. After this, the hotel staff went on strike. I shall never forget the RCN President climbing onto a table and exhorting members to take things into their own hands and get their food themselves! Politically, the pay situation led to an emergency motion, and a marathon 2-hour debate culminated in a telegram to Mrs Castle demanding an immediate meeting.

Mrs Castle agreed to meet us, and a few weeks later a delegation led by the RCN President presented her with a document *The State of Nursing*, which Mrs Castle described in the subsequent House of Commons debate on the NHS as 'one of the most poignant and impressive documents I have ever read'. Meanwhile, 2000 nurses marched with banners from Cavendish Square to Trafalgar Square. I remember standing on the lions' pedestal with megaphone in hand exhorting the crowds to action. We demanded an independent enquiry into nurses' pay and conditions, and we issued an ultimatum: if this was not granted within 21 days all RCN members would resign from the NHS, and the RCN would set up a national nursing agency to 'sell them back' to the NHS on our own terms. In Council we had discussed this proposition at length, but I for one never believed it was feasible. Fortunately we did not have to implement the threat because Mrs Castle agreed to set up an enquiry to be chaired by Lord Halsbury. There had already been sporadic strikes by the other unions. We held the line against industrial action, and were vindicated when Halsbury wrote:

Before we began our enquiry and on occasion during the course of it, a limited amount of industrial action was taken in support of the pay claim by a few groups of nurses. As an independent body we considered whether we should suspend our inquiry in the light of this action which at best was unhelpful. We want to make clear that the pressure which the industrial action was designed to create has not influenced our recommendations in any way.

The Halsbury Report gave us a 33% pay rise, but it did not stop the continuing industrial disputes, which eventually caused the downfall of the Labour government in 1979.

Reviewing the RCN membership structure

In 1973 the RCN Council initiated a review of the membership structure facilitated by the Tavistock Institute of Human Relations. The Tavistock team recommended that the whole membership should be invited to participate actively in the exercise, and in 1974 'Operation Grassroots' began. Nine regional 'talkabouts' involving over 1000 members were held across the country. Delegates were briefed to report back to their branches and sections and to continue the discussions. At the meeting of the RRB in March a whole day was devoted to discussion. The annual report carried the statement 'The beginning of a new era for the RCN with the launching of an exercise in membership participation which will lead to the development of a membership structure determined by members for members' and commented 'there will be a membership structure that has evolved because of the wishes of the members; not something imposed, but the result of a participative enterprise'. How I wish that the same could be said of the review that took place in the years following 2005.

Under the Tavistock proposals, RCN Branches were replaced by Centres. The potential membership of a Centre included all RCN members living in an area, ideally the area coterminous with the new area health authorities, which meant they were much larger than the former branches and were unrelated to workplaces. Centres had a great deal of autonomy in deciding their own activities, which included professional issues as well as workplace issues.

The members also made it clear that they wanted to retain the national network of specialist interest groups that had developed during the 1960s alongside the geographically-defined Branches – the beginning of what later became the RCN Forums. Alongside my Council role I maintained my special interest in community nursing through the Society of Primary Health Care Nursing. Three associations – the Association of Nursing Management, the Association of Nursing Education, and the Association of Nursing Practice – were established. These were soon to be followed by the Association of Nursing Students. Each association had an elected executive committee, the chair of which had a seat on Council. The Association of Nursing Students was particularly interesting because it gave students a real voice in the organisation and full voting membership of the RRB. Its leaders often went on to stellar careers in top positions in the NHS.

The key feature of this structure was the linkages between the Forums and the Associations and Societies in such a way that all the different entities had a direct link to the Council and its committees, which were where policies were agreed. This bottom-up approach ensured that the policies developed reflected the priorities and expertise of the grassroots members, and encouraged membership motivation and engagement.

The new structure, and in particular the creation of the Professional Nursing Department headed by David Rye, supported a flowering of the professional work of the RCN. A team of expert nurse advisers included some of the most talented and creative nurses of their day – Ray Rowden and later Richard Wells for oncology nursing, Paul Lloyd for mental health, Ainna Fawcett-Henesy for primary healthcare, Alan Parrish for learning disabilities nursing, and Sue Burr for paediatric nursing. Each officer was secretary to a Section and/or an Association and acted as an expert professional adviser and consultant in that specialist field, working closely with recognised nurse leaders in the field. They also provided a link with other departments including Press and Public Relations and the Labour Relations Department, which dealt with members' employment problems.

RCN Fellowships

In 1976 the RCN celebrated its 60th birthday. There were celebrations at all levels in the organisation, including two visits from royal patrons. One important development was the establishment of RCN Fellowships. The Fellowships are seen as the highest honour that the RCN can bestow, and are specifically focussed on the individual's 'outstanding contribution to the science and art of nursing' (the first purpose of the RCN as set out in its charter), as opposed to service to the RCN (for which the RCN Award of Merit was later established). I was proud to be elected as Fellow in 1982 for my work in the field of health visiting.

The Fellowship scheme has, however, had something of a chequered history that is documented in the booklet *Celebrating Excellence*, produced to celebrate its 30th anniversary in 2006. The first Fellows were clear about their role: in a residential seminar in 1980 – a glittering occasion held in Leeds Castle and opened by HRH Princess Margaret – they considered their role and the contribution they could make to the College as a corporate body. The Fellows agreed that they should act as a 'professional think tank' to the organisation, and in particular to the Council. They saw the system for the award of Fellowships as a matter for peer review by the Fellows themselves, which is how fellowships in most other professional associations are determined. The Council was suspicious of what it saw as a self-perpetuating elite, however, and changed the awarding committee to a Council committee with no representation from existing Fellows. Council was also suspicious of 'intellectual' achievements, especially when, as happened sometimes in the early years, the award of a Fellowship coincided with the award of a PhD. Several attempts were made to find a way of including the Fellows in the policy-making machinery, without much success. There was just one further seminar like the Leeds Castle event: a conference held in 1986 on the theme of justice. Other than the proceedings of these two meetings, the think-tank that I had hoped would be a useful resource for policy development never materialised.

The later Fellows themselves have been ambivalent about their role. I was elected Fellow in 1982 and when I was elected Convener in 1997 I badly wanted the Fellows to return to the original concept, and to become more like the American Academy of Nursing, which was at that time part of the American Nurses Association (it is now an independent organisation affiliated to the American Nurses Association). The Academy's mission is 'to serve the public and the nursing profession by advancing health policy and practice through the generation, synthesis, and dissemination of nursing knowledge'. Fellowship of the American Academy of Nursing is regarded as a high honour in the USA, and I was very proud indeed to be elected Fellow in 2010 – one of very few nurses from outside the USA. I believed, and still believe, that the RCN Fellows have a huge amount of experience and expertise and that they could and should act as a professional think-tank. Following my election as Convener I undertook a survey to find out what Fellows wanted, and was bitterly disappointed by the result: almost half saw their Fellowship as merely a reward for past achievements with no ongoing commitment to the organisation; they did not see themselves as a corporate body, and did not want to be involved in any activities. American Academy of Nursing literature, in contrast, specifically states that 'Invitation to fellowship is more than recognition of one's accomplishments within the nursing profession. Academy fellows also have a responsibility to contribute their time and energies to the Academy, and to engage with other health care leaders outside the Academy in transforming America's health care system'.

Despite general ambivalence, I was determined to try to do something to improve the role of RCN Fellow. In 1999 the centenary meeting of the ICN was to be held in London, and I knew that leaders of the American Nurses Association and the American Academy of Nursing would be there. Two of these leaders, Vernice Ferguson and Norma Lang, whom I knew well, were Fellows both of the American Academy of Nursing and (Honorary) Fellows of the RCN. I therefore got the idea of having a joint meeting that would include presentations on the roles of the Fellows in the two organisations as well as debate on the nursing issues of the day. Vernice chaired, Joyce Fitzpatrick (then President of the American Academy) and I spoke on the roles of Fellows, and Norma and David Rye led the debates on nursing issues. The proceedings were published in a special issue of *Nursing Leadership Forum*, a journal that Joyce edited. The meeting was a success, but my views on the development of the Fellows were not popular. In the election for Convener a few months later I was voted out.

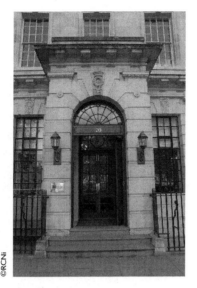

RCN Head Office, 20 Cavendish Square, London

CHAPTER 9: THE GOLDEN YEARS

Looking back, I think the late 1970s and the 1980s were the heyday of the RCN, in particular of its work as a professional association. One indicator is the string of publications produced by the Forums and Societies on a range of professional issues. The members of the working groups were always listed by name, and since they were recognised experts in their field, this gave the documents credibility.

Work on standards – a major consideration for any professional association – was also carried out. Throughout the 1970s the RCN became increasingly concerned and vocal about standards of nursing care. In 1978 the Council established a working committee, later formalised as the Standing Committee on Standards of Nursing Care, of which I was a member. The working committee was chaired by Dame Sheila Quinn, who brought to the work her extensive international knowledge, including the work being undertaken by the American Nurses Association to develop statements of standards for nursing using the structure–process–outcome framework first developed by Avedis Donabedian and applied to nursing by Norma Lang.

129

A first report, *Standards of Nursing Care*, was published in 1980, and a second, *Towards Standards*, in 1981. I took what I had learned back to my 'day job' as Senior Nurse (Research) in West Berkshire and, with Helen Kendall, began to develop a programme of standard statements based on the American Nurses Association format. This was the work that in 1985 Alison Kitson found, and which she developed into Dynamic Standard Setting System (referred to as the DySSSy system).

The DySSSy system was a huge success. It spread throughout the UK and several other countries, especially in Scandinavia. In the UK teaching materials were prepared, workshops were held around the country, and each RCN Forum produced a document specifying standards for their own specialty. The key features of the DySSSy system were:

- Small groups of nurses working together with a facilitator to set standards relevant to their own area of practice
- A standardised format for writing statements, based on the three dimensions of structure, process and outcome
- An indexing system that enabled standards set in one specialty or clinical area to be related to similar standards set elsewhere
- A means of ensuring that the standards set were agreed by the relevant manager
- A means of ensuring that the standards were used in practice and regularly reviewed.

An important feature of the system was the empowerment of nurses to take control of their own practice and to set their own standards in fields in which they were expert. The RCN still claims standards of practice as a major concern, but no longer uses the DySSSy system. The RCN no longer sets standards, but instead endorses, where relevant, standards set by other organisations. The ideology of empowering nurses to set their own standards has disappeared.

Throughout the 1980s much of the RCN's work focused on the development of nursing practice, advanced nursing practice, clinical career structures, and an issue central to all of these – the nurse's accountability. 'Accountability in Nursing' was the theme of the Fellows' Leeds Castle seminar in 1980; summaries of the presentations given by several distinguished Fellows from UK and other counties are included in the published report. In the Society of Primary Health Care Nursing, triggered by the publicity being given at the time to child abuse, health visitors were increasingly concerned about their accountability. From a series of weekend workshops, the Society's Health Visiting Advisory Group, which I chaired, produced two documents: *Thinking about Health Visiting* (1983), which raised several issues for discussion, and *Accountability in Health Visiting* (1984), which expanded the chapter in *Thinking about Health Visiting* that had produced most debate in the seminars that followed the first document. We developed a model for understanding accountability that can be used in any field: it shows that accountability is always for something (the charge) to someone (nurses are accountable to several different people for different charges), and that accountability requires the ability (including resources), the giving and acceptance of responsibility, and the authority to carry out the charge. Later, when Ainna Fawcett-Henesy, who was at this time the RCN's Nurse Adviser for Primary Health Care, became the Regional Adviser on Nursing and Midwifery for Europe at the WHO, I was invited to expand this in a paper for the WHO Ministerial Conference on Nursing held in Munich in 2000.

Chair of RRB

In 1978 I was elected Chair of the RCN Representative Body (RRB), later to be renamed and now universally known as RCN Congress. During my first year as Chair, the meeting was held in Guernsey. As it was such a lovely location where Roger had enjoyed many childhood holidays, he and our two children, then aged 7 and 10, came with me. We went out a week early for a family holiday. For the first time, on my initiative, we organised a crèche for members' children, so several members and staff also brought their youngsters along; the 13 children had a wonderful time, and now the crèche is an established facility at Congress.

It was fortunate that we did go early, because on the day before Congress was due to start, the fog came down. Since at that time Guernsey had no facilities for aeroplanes to land in fog, travel to Guernsey from the mainland was impossible. The last members eventually arrived, a day late, often having been diverted through France or Dublin. Luggage was lost, so Marks & Spencer did a roaring trade in underwear and new suits. Of the guest speakers scheduled to speak at the pre-RRB conference on the theme 'Standards', only the Chairman, David Jacobs, arrived – after a sleepless all-night boat trip from Southampton. This disaster was, however, turned into a triumph as the gap was filled by speakers from within the organisation, who gave a magnificent performance. It was a turning point in the developing self-confidence of nursing and the RCN.

After a long and exhausting day, I had to prepare for the RRB meeting that began the next morning. I had had no pre-meeting briefing, although I

131

had talked with my predecessor Sam Richards, for whose wise guidance I was grateful. All my predecessors as Chair of the RRB had senior work roles, with secretaries whom they could use to support their RCN roles, whereas I was still in a junior post without any back-up resources to call upon. The only tools I had were the agenda as printed in the pull-out supplement in the *Nursing Standard*, and a copy of the constitution and standing orders. General Secretary Catherine Hall sat at my right hand with her own pile of papers, however, ready to fill the deficit.

The Agenda Committee, which in those days consisted mainly of the senior staff, was scheduled to meet after dinner in the General Secretary's hotel suite. The staff, who to be fair, had worked tirelessly to make the day a success in spite of the difficulties, wanted only to relax over a few drinks, which were available in plentiful supply. I knew I had to keep my wits about me, and by midnight, when I could see that I was going to have to rely on my own resources, I left the meeting and repaired to my own room to prepare as best I could. I had a system of index cards, each of which set out what I was to do in the event of, for example, procedural motions or a card vote. I spent the next 2 hours going over them and the agenda items until I fell asleep.

Following the opening formalities, we had 47 resolutions and 'matters for discussion', plus any emergency motions that might be submitted during the week. In those days the agenda was themed, with sections on general issues (seven motions), health service practice and policy (nine motions), salaries and conditions of service (11 motions), professional policy (eight motions), nursing education (nine motions), and RCN organisation and membership (three motions) on different days. It is interesting to note how many of the issues discussed nowadays were on the agenda then – abuse of alcohol and tobacco, resources for community nursing services, violence in accident and emergency departments, car allowances. Among the most significant, in the light of later developments, were a matter for discussion on the implications of industrial action and one about the need for 'an evaluation of the present membership structure with particular reference to the position of associations and specialist societies in relation to local centres'.

The issue of the week, however, was the motion submitted by Council that 'the College should proceed forthwith to make application to the Trades Union Congress for affiliation to that Congress'. The motion was overwhelmingly carried, so following our meeting a series of meetings was held around the country to explain the implications of affiliation in preparation for the anticipated vote. Although I had not been able to express any view during the debate at the RRB meeting, I was now able to present the RRB position – which in fact accorded with my personal view – that we should affiliate. Trevor Clay, who was about to succeed Catherine Hall as General Secretary, was also in favour. There was much debate about the costs, which would have been considerable, but my view was that we really had no choice: the government was limiting pay negotiations to TUC-affiliated organisations only, and if we wanted to continue to be there in the corridors of power we had to join. There was no certainty that the TUC would accept an application from us; the other health service unions could be expected to oppose our application. There were considerable behind-the-scenes negotiations with the TUC leaders to try to avoid such humiliation. In the event, in May 1979 the general election ousted the Labour government and brought in the Conservative government led by Margaret Thatcher, which immediately disempowered the TUC. Affiliation was no longer necessary, and the RCN membership ballot rejected the proposal. The issue has been debated at RRB several times since, but as the power of the TUC gradually diminished, the RCN membership support for affiliation has also declined.

Congress in those days was less sophisticated but much more fun than it is now. Debates really were debates, with speakers using standing orders (as I had been doing for several years) for points of order and procedural motions; there was even one congress 'character', who came to be called 'Morrison Point of Order'. The technology was primitive – no electronic management of microphones or for voting. To limit speaking time, a member of staff sat on my left with a clock and a board on which were mounted three bulbs, each with a manually-operated on/off switch. When the green light was on, the speaker could speak; when the green light was replaced by the yellow light, the speaker had 1 minute left; at 30 seconds the red light was flashed on and off until time-up was signalled by the red light staying on. On one occasion when I felt a speaker was droning on for too long, I leaned across to the timekeeper and whispered: 'Give him a quick flash!' Unfortunately the microphones picked up my whisper and the whole audience collapsed in laughter.

As now, we raised money for good causes. One year at Bournemouth we had an early-morning sponsored splash, and on one famous occasion I wandered through the exhibition with my mouth sealed by duct tape and holding a bucket. As now, there were parties every night, and I prided myself on putting in an appearance at them all. The students' party was always fancy dress, and I have some wonderful photos with James Smith in a nightshirt and Dave Dawes dressed as a Roman soldier. The 'Welsh night' usually ended with a singsong round the piano, and at the last one under my chairmanship I famously performed a solo item:

Chairman's lament (based on Annie's song in Oklahoma)

It ain't so much a question of not knowing what to do
I've knowed what's right and wrong since I was 10.
I've heard a lot of stories, though I know that they ain't true,
About those prissy folks in RCN.
I know I should keep quiet and just sit
But when they start to argue I forgit!

I'm just a girl who can't say no, I'm in a terrible fix.
I always say come on let's go, just when I ought to say nix.
When the bar is open or the party's on
I know I ought to say I'm off to bed;
But as soon as someone says 'Come on'
I somehow sort of go right off my head.

I'm just a fool at RRB
I cant be prissy and quaint, I ain't the type that can faint,
How can I be what I ain't
I can't say no.

What you going to do when the Minister gets shirty
And starts to play dirty,
What you going to do?
Supposing he says that your stance he applauds it
But the country can't afford it,
What you going to do?
Supposing there's a speaker gotta speak now
And he's gotta speak now or die,
What you gonna do when he flashes his card –
Turn a blind eye?

I'm just a girl who can't say no, can't even say what I'd like,
I have to sit and bite my tongue when I'd rather be standing at a mike.
For while I act refined and cool,
Asitting 'tween the Dame and dearest Sam,
When I think of pay and that ol' Rule
The standing orders all of them I'd ban!

I can't resist a good debate, especially at RRB,
So wait until Bournemouth next year, you ain't heard the last I fear,
I can't say no!

Before the introduction of the deafening disco noise, however, the parties were used for serious lobbying. RRB really was a mechanism by which grassroots members directly influenced policy: our agenda included between 40 and 50 motions, and if any dropped off the end because of lack of time they were directly remitted to Council for discussion there. Nowadays Congress is heavily stage-managed with, in my view, more of an eye to press and public relations than to policy development. There are outside speakers and rarely more than a dozen items for debate, and speakers come to the microphone to deliver speeches prepared before they have heard any debate. What it has gained in sophistication it has lost in spontaneity.

The 'winter of discontent'

Soon after I was elected Chair of RRB the RCN was caught up in the 1978/9 'winter of discontent' in which public sector workers challenged the government's pay policy with industrial action including strikes. The Staff Side of the Nurses and Midwives' Whitley Council demanded that nurses' pay be restored to the level achieved after the 1974 Halsbury award, and the RCN launched a pay campaign with the title 'Pay not Peanuts'. When Prime Minister James Callaghan refused to meet the Staff Side, anger exploded and the RCN Council, of which I was a member by virtue of being Chair of the RRB, decided to set up an action committee to pursue the pay claim. I was elected Chairman. Feelings were running very high; for the first time RCN members were actively discussing strike action, and in particular whether or not to change Rule 12, which forbade RCN members from taking industrial action. On 11 December the Staff Side sent a telegram to the Prime Minister drawing attention to the nurses' mounting anger and frustration and requesting an urgent meeting. In the continuing absence of a positive response, the Action Committee recommended two things: first, that at its meeting scheduled to take place on 11 January, the Council should call an extraordinary general meeting for the purpose of amending Rule 12; and second that the RCN should convene a national protest meeting to take place on 18 January, to be followed by a mass lobby of Parliament. Council agreed. Meanwhile other unions were planning industrial action, in some cases including all-out strike.

The national protest meeting took place despite coinciding with a national rail strike. Some 2300 RCN members packed into Central Hall

Westminster, where they were addressed by representatives of the main political parties, the General Secretary, and myself. The atmosphere was electric. The politicians were fiercely heckled. Catherine Hall and I spoke to tumultuous applause and a standing ovation. Over the years I have made many speeches and received many standing ovations, but I think none has been more impassioned than this one:

Enough is enough. What more can we do? What we are asking for seems to me eminently sensible and reasonable. Firstly the restoration in 1979 cash figures, of principles which were established by an independent inquiry, agreed by both sides of the Whitley Council and by Government – by everybody – only 4 years ago. Secondly a mechanism to make these principles permanent, so that we no longer have to suffer nor to inflict on the public the quadrennial purge that Miss Hall has described. Is this so difficult to understand that a decision has to be so long delayed? Is this so unreasonable? In my naivety I believed that our society was in essence a civilised society, a just society, in which a reasonable case would always be heard, and if the case was sound it would be supported.... So why are we here? We are here because we have learnt the hard way – by experience – that a just case is not enough.... For each one of us here there are ten of our colleagues at work, providing the service to which we are committed. Some will have walked to work today because there are no trains. Some will be considering how to care for incontinent old ladies when, on Monday, there may be no laundry. Up in the North West health visitors will be trying to explain to confused young mothers why they must boil the water their children are to drink....

This [industrial action] is the course of action which we would propose. We hope that it will not be necessary, that this plan will never be implemented. But let the Government be in no doubt that if it is implemented it will bite in the two places where it hurts the Government most – in its pocket at the Treasury, and in public confidence, its electoral image. And let the Government be in no doubt: if this action must be taken, it will be taken. If this is what the government requires, then that is what we must do.

The Action Committee had been tasked by the RCN Council with developing a plan for industrial action to be implemented if the Extraordinary General Meeting voted to change Rule 12. We struggled over what we could do within the principles Council had agreed. These were that any action must reflect professional policies, must minimise the effect on patients, must be practicable and must be visible (i.e. must be newsworthy and attract publicity). I agonised then, and have done so on many occasions since, about nurses and industrial action. The RCN Congress has debated motions supporting industrial action several times since 1979, and all such motions have been rejected by large majorities. In 1981, when we were in the throes of yet another pay campaign and were again under pressure to change Rule 12, I wrote in my monthly column in *The Health Supplement*:

'The tragedy is that even if such action did achieve a larger than average pay award it would be a pyrrhic victory. Trust is the essence of the nurse–patient relationship, and once that trust is broken on either an individual or a societal level things can never be quite the same again.... Does this government really want to go down in history as the one which finally forced nurses past the breaking point?'

Some months after the events of 1979, when the General Nursing Council (a predecessor of the Nursing and Midwifery Council) issued a statement that any nurse who took industrial action would 'have a case to answer' for professional misconduct, I wrote an article in the *Nursing Mirror* under the title 'The right to strike'. I argued that although nurses, like other employees, have the right to strike and should not be deprived of it, they should decline to exercise it because to do so would conflict with the responsibilities that they accepted in choosing to become nurses. I argued that the 'professional misconduct' lay not in the particular action but in the 'putting patients at risk'. Limitation of services such as those identified by the Action Committee would constitute industrial action only if it were done in pursuit of an industrial dispute and not in pursuit of protecting patients or securing standards of care. In other words, the definition depends on the motivation and not on the tasks themselves. I still agonise over the argument that action that may harm the individual but benefits the group is justifiable; action is justifiable if a few patients suffer now in the interest of saving greater numbers of patients in the future. As recently as 2011, in response to further pressure from some members to support a planned public sector National Day of Action, the Council decided not to ballot members, but reaffirmed its position that although they were empowered to initiate industrial action, they would not authorise any action that was 'detrimental to the wellbeing or interests of patients'. Way back in 1979, as a result of the work of the Action Committee, I had already come to the conclusion that there was nothing we could do that would be effective but not harm patients: promoting the Action Committee's plan when I knew in my heart that it would not work was hard.

In the event it was not necessary to implement the plan. When the EGM was held on 26 February there was a dramatic change of mood: the motion to abolish Rule 12 was overwhelmingly rejected. Why was there such a dramatic change? The answer is simple: between the two meetings, other health service unions took industrial action including all-out strike action, and for the first time nurses saw the reality of what it did to patients. Laundries stopped work so patients languished in wet and dirty sheets; kitchens stopped work so patients had no hot food; ambulances had to be manned by policemen, who did not have the skills of the paramedics they were replacing; bodies piled up in temporary mortuaries; and rubbish piled up everywhere. At the RRB in April, James Smith, who was then District Nursing Officer in Brent, vividly described how patients had suffered as his district was 'crippled'.

An unexpected election result

The debates about industrial action continue to surface from time to time. In 1981 the debate produced one very unexpected result. That year was the first time the president of the RCN was directly elected by the whole membership; previously presidents had been elected by the Council from among the Council's own members. There were four candidates: Sheila Quinn, Sheila Collins, Sam Richards (all experienced and well known RCN leaders) and a totally unknown member from Wales called Marion Morgan. Marion was at this time the Chief Nursing Officer of Powys Health Authority, in which role I knew her slightly through my own Welsh links. Against everyone's expectation, Marion was elected. At our post-election orientation meeting for the new honorary officers (I was there by virtue of being Chair of the Representative Body) Marion confided to me how she had come to be nominated. She said she had been ill in bed when she received a telephone call from the Chairman of her local RCN Branch asking her if she was willing to 'stand for President'. Marion assumed that this meant President of the Branch – the most senior nurse in the area often took this role, and Marion was popular with her staff. Feeling very unwell, she just said yes and went back to sleep. Having once been nominated, she said she felt she could not back out. But how did someone so completely unknown get elected? One reason could be that the three well-known candidates split the vote, but I think there was another reason. We were yet again in the middle of a pay campaign and more debate about industrial action, and just at the time when the voting papers went out, Marion had published an article in the *Nursing Standard* in which she had written that she would support her staff if they decided to take industrial action – a view very popular with grassroots members as opposed to the 'establishment'. Marion was delighted to be elected but did not find the role easy, partly because of her inexperience of the RCN, but also because her employing authority was not willing to give the support that such a demanding role required. Marion was, however, valiantly supported by Sheila Quinn, who had been elected Deputy President and was duly elected President in the next election.

Trevor Clay's reign

In 1979 Trevor Clay became Deputy General Secretary, and then, when Catherine Hall retired to become Chairman of the newly-established UK Central Council for Nursing Midwifery and Health Visiting (UKCC) in 1982, became General Secretary. Trevor often said that he 'burned for nursing', and it showed. Trevor was a charismatic leader, a skilful speaker, well-known nationally and internationally (he became a member of the ICN's Board of Directors). The 8 years of his reign were, in my view, when the RCN reached its zenith. Membership grew at a rate faster than ever before or since. These years included the 'Pay Not Peanuts' and the 'Bridge that Gap' pay campaigns, the establishment of the Pay Review Body, the Griffiths Report, the 'RCN

Trevor Clay with Dame Sheila Quinn at ICN Congress

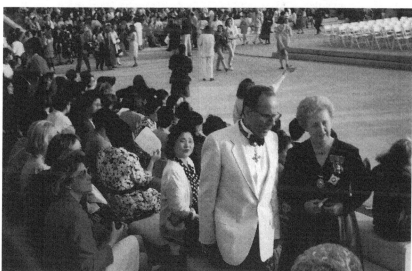

Nurse Alert' campaign, and clinical grading. Alongside these trade union activities were major professional activities including the Commission on Nursing Education (the Judge Report), the work on developing standards, the submissions and responses to the Cumberlege review of community nursing and Project 2000. Internally there was continuing review of the membership structure, the development of the Professional Nursing Department (led by David Rye), the establishment of the Parliamentary Office (initially led by Neil Stewart, formerly President of the National Union of Students), the expansion of the Press and PR Department (led by Alison Dunn) including the development of the *Nursing Standard* into a weekly journal and the establishment of Scutari Projects Ltd, the transformation of the RRB into RCN Congress (led by Brian French), and completion of the refurbishment of our headquarters (with its new address as 20 Cavendish Square). At this time there was, in fact, a total rebranding of the RCN as a professional association and a trade union. It was an exciting time.

Trevor was a committed trade unionist, but he was just as committed to professionalism, and is credited with the first description of the RCN as a 'professional trade union', a concept he discussed in his book, *Nurses: Power and Politics* published in 1987. He was also a 'membership man'. Unlike any general secretary before or since, Trevor came to the appointment with a track record of engagement in the RCN as an activist at all levels. He had been a branch chairman, an active member of the (then) Ward and Departmental Section, a popular speaker at RRB, Chair of the Association of Nursing Management and a member of the Council. He understood members and the delicate balance of power between members and staff. He used to hold what came to be called 'kiln dinners' (a pun derived from his name) with the honorary officers at Cavendish Square. At these dinners, when we got as far as the dessert, he would pull out from his inside jacket pocket a little silver notebook and a pencil with the words: 'I've had an idea which I just want to run past you'. Of course we knew that he was about to tell us about plans he had already formulated, but he never promoted a plan or made a major decision before first discussing it with us and securing our support. Sadly, he suffered for several years from emphysema and in 1989 was forced to retire. One of the worst moments of my life was when, as RCN President, I had to take the platform at the opening of Congress 1994 to report his death.

The Clegg Report

By 1981 we were in the throes of yet another pay campaign, this time as the result of the Standing Commission on Pay Comparability chaired by

Professor Hugh Clegg. Somewhat wearily I wrote in my column in *The Health Supplement* on 4 December:

I do not relish the thought of another nurses' pay campaign and I do not know of any nurse who does. It is only two years since the last one, and the wounds of that battle have not healed. I find the experience of "parading my poverty before the public" as the Guardian recently put it, deeply humiliating. I have more important things to do with my time – such as nursing patients – than addressing campaign meetings and distributing leaflets. But what do nurses have to do to achieve the improvement which everyone already agrees is just and necessary?'

The pay award that followed the Clegg Report was different from its predecessors in that it was very divisive internally because it changed the traditional differentials between the various grades of staff; in particular it gave greater increases to the clinical grades than to tutors and managers. In an article in the *Nursing Mirror* I supported this approach, but incurred the wrath of nurse tutors when I wrote:

We cannot have it both ways. If we want nurse tutors to be comparable with [further education] lecturers then we must change our crazy system of recruiting and training them, and tutors must give up the cloistered cosiness of schools of nursing and face the intellectual challenge of research based multi-disciplinary teaching.

The phrase 'cloistered cosiness' produced a quite hysterical reaction in the correspondence columns, and nurse teachers never forgave me. The Editor, Mark Allen, wrote to me privately: 'I am appalled that it seems to have sparked off such a hysterical reaction. It seems to me extraordinary that some people are incapable of taking part in a cool and reasoned debate. When nurses become so small-minded I feel like packing my bags.' I received several private letters of support, including one from Christine Hancock, who wrote: 'Your phrase "cloistered cosiness" is glorious – don't ever regret it.'

My key message, however, is as true today as it was then: 'The result is that we spend so much energy scratching out one another's eyes that we have none left to fight the common (external) enemy. United we might stand, but divided they rule.' The dispute rumbled on until eventually the Review Body for Nursing Staff, Midwives, Health Visitors and Professions Allied to Medicine was established in 1983. The battles over nurses' pay continue, but there have been no more of the kind I experienced throughout the 70s.

The Griffiths report

The next big challenge of Trevor's reign was the publication of the Griffiths Report in 1983. Since 1974 health services at local level had been managed by multidisciplinary teams consisting of a community physician, a hospital consultant and a GP (chosen by the hospital doctors and GPs), a chief nurse, a treasurer, and an administrator. Decisions were made by consensus, with any one member of the team having power of veto. The chief nurse managed the whole of the nursing service and enjoyed considerable power, not only as a result of the power of veto but because she managed and controlled the budget for nursing, which, because of the numbers of nurses, was the largest element in the total budget. This was not compatible with Mrs Thatcher's new business ideology; she invited Roy Griffiths, the Managing Director of Sainsbury's, to review the management arrangements of the NHS. There was no scope for consultation, no committee or commission to which to submit evidence as would have happened before; the recommendations of the Griffiths report were expressed in a letter to Norman Fowler, Secretary of State for Health, and Mrs Thatcher accepted them for immediate implementation.

The new arrangement was the introduction of general management. Nurses were not mentioned in the report except in the much-quoted remark that: 'If Florence Nightingale were carrying her lamp around the corridors of the NHS today she would almost certainly be searching for the people in charge.' At a subsequent conference I retorted: 'If Florence Nightingale were carrying her lamp around the corridors of the NHS today, she would almost certainly be in charge.' Roy Griffiths said that he never intended to disempower nurses, but nurses were caught in the crossfire. At a dinner held at the RCN some time later at which I sat next to him, he protested: 'Don't blame me, I never implemented the bloody thing.' Certainly he did not intend the loss of the chief nursing officer, matron and the ward sister that followed as a consequence of the implementation of general management right down to ward level.

The effect of the Griffiths report, whether intended or not, was to wipe out nursing management. With it went much of nursing's power for more than a decade. The RCN mounted a vigorous publicity campaign with posters carrying slogans such as 'Why is Britain's nursing being run by people who don't know their coccyx from their humerus?' One of the most powerful said: 'You're in hospital. It's dark. You're all alone, surrounded by strangers. You're worried in case something happens. And you're the nurse.'

The Cumberledge review

Hot on the heels of the Griffiths report came the Cumberlege Review of Community Nursing Services. Julia Cumberlege (later Baroness Cumberlege) was known as a prominent Conservative Party activist, wife of a wealthy Sussex farmer, and Chairperson of Brighton Health Authority. We were still smarting from the wounds of the Griffiths review and terrified that this review would follow the same pattern, so the Society of Primary Care Nursing set up a small team – which included myself, Deborah Henessey and Barbara Stillwell, supported by Ainna Fawcett-Henesy, the nurse adviser for primary care – and we decided to take the initiative: we invited her to meet us.

As Julia walked through the door she appeared to confirm my worst fears and all my prejudices about female Conservative politicians: she oozed elegance, wearing a beautiful pale blue cashmere twinset with a magnificent string of pearls. In the event I could not have been more wrong about her. When we asked whether she would be willing to receive evidence from us, she readily agreed with a steely gaze and the words: 'I have no wish to give birth to a stillborn child.'

We prepared a detailed document setting out our views about the future of community nursing, including our proposals for the introduction of nurse prescribing and for the development of the nurse practitioner in primary care (the role that Barbara Stillwell was pioneering). We welcomed the report *Neighbourhood Nursing: a Focus for Care*, which adopted our proposals, and began two decades of work on getting them implemented.

Despite our work, the report was rejected by the Government, largely because of the concerted opposition of the GPs, who saw the increased autonomy proposed for nurses as a threat to their own authority and control. In particular, they fought against the proposal that practice nurses, whom they directly employed and therefore controlled, should work for the district health authorities alongside other members of the community nursing team. Sadly, many practice nurses agreed, largely because traditional nursing management was regarded as rigid and bureaucratic compared with the 'freedom' of the private arrangements negotiated by individual GPs. We were concerned because this 'freedom' meant that many practice nurses had no training for the work being delegated to them (for which the GPs were paid), there was no supervision or system of monitoring standards of practice, and contracts of employment where they existed were inadequate. Quite apart from the external opposition, the debate within the RCN was vitriolic; many practice nurses attacked the RCN's position, and some resigned, wooed by the offer of associate membership of the Royal College of General Practitioners. At one conference, Ainna famously remarked that she 'knew of only one other profession where men are paid for the work of women'. Not for the first or last time nurses were divided on the issue of professional autonomy vis-à-vis subservience to doctors. It took a long time, but eventually the outcome of the struggle was positive: the best of the practice nurse leaders came together to put their own house in order and the RCN Practice Nurses Forum became one of the most active membership groups within the RCN.

Julia was in my view treated disgracefully both by the medical profession and, under their pressure, by the government, which published her report only as an appendix to their Green Paper on primary care. Julia was not one to take rejection lying down, however; she stood her ground and met the opposition head on. In collaboration with us, she organised and funded from her own private means a series of roadshows and seminars around the country to promote the *Neighbourhood Nursing* report and fight for the implementation of its proposals. As we travelled around the country and I got to know her, I developed an enormous respect and admiration for her, which has continued ever since. Working with the RCN, she kept up the campaign for nurse prescribing for the next 20 years, using all her political skills and opportunities, from 1990 as a life peer and from 1992 as a junior Health Minister, until these proposals were implemented. In 2006, 20 years on from her *Neighbourhood Nursing* report, the RCN hosted a party to celebrate the implementation of nurse prescribing. Julia continues to be a great champion of community nursing, in recognition for which she was made RCN Vice President in 1989 and an Honorary Fellow in 2010.

Nursing education

The Judge Report

While I was fully occupied with the community nursing agenda, another major agenda item was the future of nursing education. Impatient with the continuing inaction of the UKCC, which had been establishd with a commitment to review nursing education, the RCN decided to take the initiative and established its own Commission on Nursing Education under the chairmanship of Professor Harry Judge, Director of the Department of Educational Studies in the University of Oxford. Its report, *The Education of Nurses: A New Dispensation*, was published in 1985. Its proposals were radical: it rejected the apprenticeship model of hospital-based nurse training in favour of 'the wholesale shifting of the apparatus of nurse education outside the NHS'. A corollary of this move was the recommendation for full student status, with student nurses receiving a non means-tested bursary. The Judge Report recommended an integrated, modular 3-year course in which the first year would be a foundation course common to all students, followed by opportunities for specialisation but leading to a single grade of qualified nurse and a Diploma in Nursing Studies, to be followed by a period of supervised practice within a locally-provided continuing education programme.

Project 2000

At the same time as the RCN was working on the Judge Report, the UKCC had begun a series of discussion papers on topics including pre-registration specialisation and the abolition of the second-level nurse. Once again, nursing was beset by internal divisions. Harry Judge famously remarked: 'Nurses will get the education they want when they say clearly and unambiguously what they want.' The UKCC's report, *Project 2000: A New Preparation for Practice*, was published in May 1986 and it recommended:

- A 3-year programme consisting of a 2-year common foundation programme followed by a 1-year branch programme, leading to a Diploma in Higher Education and registration as a qualified nurse with the relevant branch specified in the title
- Branch programmes to include adult nursing, children's nursing, mental health nursing, learning disability nursing, and midwifery
- Second-level training (state-enrolled nursing or SEN) to be phased out
- Full student status with no contribution to rostered service
- 'Links' with the higher and further education sector.

Never has a report been so misunderstood and misrepresented. P 2000 (as it came to be called) has been unfairly blamed for all of the failings in nursing ever since. For example, it was not Project 2000 that moved nursing into the universities, it merely recommended 'links', and with further as well as higher education. Nor did it recommend that the academic level of pre-registration education should be set at degree level. Those things came several years later. Contrary to current popular belief, the proportion of time in clinical practice remained unchanged, as required by the 1977 EU Directives on nursing. Since the new-style programmes did not begin until the early 1990s, the great majority of the workforce consisted of nurses trained under the 'old' system until well past the year 2000.

Moreover, Project 2000 was a consultation document, not a mandated programme: in addition to the differences of opinion revealed before its publication, a number of changes were made between its publication in 1986 and its implementation several years later, several of which severely compromised some of its most basic aims and principles. Midwives opposed the idea of a midwifery branch and fought for, and won, direct entry to midwifery following an entirely separate programme at undergraduate level. The common foundation programme was reduced from 2 years to 1 year. Many of the compromises were the result of negotiations with the Department of Health about the perceived costs of implementation, especially the costs of replacing student labour.

The concession that made me most angry was the loss of full student status, for which the RCN had fought for more than 40 years. When it became clear that the level of the new student bursary would be lower than the level of the previous student nurse salaries, the RCN (and the other trade unions) went straight into trade union negotiation mode. Kenneth Clarke, as Secretary of State for Health, said that an increase in the bursary would require 'something in return'. It was agreed that in return student nurses would give 1000 hours of rostered service during their third year – just under half of their total clinical practice requirement. As a result, now when a student is on the ward there is understandable confusion about whether s/he is supernumerary or not, and the culture that students are part of the ward staff persists. As when the UKCC legislation was at risk in 1979, the RCN decided that disagreements over details should not be allowed to put the main thrust of the proposals at risk. Although an extensive consultation with members demonstrated several disagreements, the RCN stated that: 'There was a widespread view that this could well be a "last chance" for the profession and that disagreement over relatively minor points should not be allowed to stand in the way of unity on the fundamental issues.'

Nursing education is still a contested issue, and in my view nursing failed to use the opportunity that Project 2000 offered. In the negotiations that moved nursing education into the universities a few years later, the RCN failed to play much of a part: the deal was done between the universities' Committee of Vice Chancellors and Principals and the Department of Health's Human Resources Department. Harry Judge's remark that 'Nurses will get the education they want when they say clearly and unambiguously what they want' still holds true. To his remark I would add: 'and when the profession takes control instead of allowing government to hold it to ransom.'

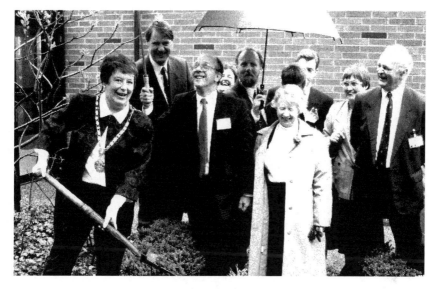

Presidential duties: planting a tree

CHAPTER 10: MADAM PRESIDENT

In 1990 I was elected President of the RCN and again in 1992 for a further term. It was undoubtedly the peak of my nursing career, but it was also the most productive period of my work within the RCN. Internally I chaired a working group with Sally Gooch, Stuart Mahon and Maureen Woods, which considered the committee structure of Council; we looked at accountability, membership access and policy making; we recommended new constitutions, with clear lines of accountability direct to Council through council member involvement on all committees, and new processes that opened up the structures to greater involvement of grassroots members. We undertook a major review of the membership entities with similar principles in mind: to facilitate membership participation, to encourage flexible working, and to develop a structure able to respond quickly to changes in membership interests and developments in nursing. We reviewed and revised the constitution and standing orders of Congress, and the remit of the Agenda Committee. I chaired the working group on the future educational function of the College and I also chaired the Research Committee. I was deeply involved in just about every aspect of the work of the RCN as a professional association and was very visible as its elected leader.

Then and now I was driven by a passionate belief that the RCN belongs to and must be run by its members. I believe that the leadership of the organisation belongs to those whom the members have elected to represent them – in particular the President, who is the only person (along with the Deputy President) elected by the whole membership. I made it my business to communicate with members at all levels, and to represent their views at every opportunity in speeches and in the media as well as in Council and its committees. Sometimes I got into trouble because I always insisted on writing my own speeches, although I took advice on which topics and angles were important.

The relationship between the president, as the elected leader, and the general secretary, as the chief executive, is particularly important. The RCN model differs from other trade unions in which the general secretary is elected, and from some other nursing organisations (e.g. the American Nurses Association and Sigma Theta Tau International) in which the elected president is the recognised head of the organisation supported by the chief executive. I believe that, properly managed, the RCN model is a good model. Of all the general secretaries that I have worked with (five in all), the one that managed it best was Trevor Clay. Sadly, in recent years the model has been eroded, to the extent that the chief executive leads as well as manages the organisation: the presidential role is now much less visible.

I believe in the distinction between management and leadership. In a membership organisation it is the job of the chief executive to manage the organisation, but the leadership rests with the elected leader – in the case of the RCN, the RCN President. In my 20 years as a member of Council, and for 4 years as Deputy President, I had worked with several RCN presidents, and I was clear about what the role entailed. I saw an important part of the role as carrying and articulating the organisational vision, ensuring a high profile, being fully involved in internal and external activities, and often acting as spokesperson to the media. If the RCN mantra is that it is 'the voice of nursing', I saw myself as 'the voice of the RCN'.

The time that I was able to give to the role was made possible by an agreement reached by Council some years earlier that if a president was also in fulltime employment, his/her employer could be 'compensated' for up to 2 days a week by payment by the RCN of up to two-fifths of his/her salary. I was the first president to enjoy this privilege, and I certainly could not have undertaken the role without it. By this time our children were 'grown and flown' and Roger was thoroughly supportive. Without Roger's full and loving support, I could not have done what I did. In addition to days away speaking at conferences and representing the RCN at various national and international events, two or three times a week after working a full day at the university I would drive from Enfield to headquarters for briefing meetings before arriving home late in the evening.

Continuing the primary care agenda

My work on community nursing and primary health care within the RCN was part of a wider agenda. All over the world primary care was moving to the top of the health policy agenda, somewhat belatedly reflected in the UK Green Paper on Primary Care and the Cumberlege review. The problem was that the UK government did not adopt the definition of 'primary health care' as set out in the Declaration of Alma Ata. In 1987 in our response to the Green Paper, Consultation on Primary Health Care initiated by the UK Health Departments, we wrote:

The RCN regrets that the Green Paper, in spite of its title Primary Health Care makes no reference to the concept of primary health care which the UK government endorsed in 1978 in the Declaration of Alma Ata. It focuses instead on the much narrower definition of primary medical care as provided through existing general practitioner services [...]. The RCN wishes to stress that primary health care is far wider than just primary medical care, and is based on a multi-disciplinary and multisectoral approach to meeting people's basic health needs; primary health care services should provide comprehensive first level and continuing healthcare to people at local level through an integrated network of services.

The RCN continued to promote the Alma Ata definition and philosophy, and in particular the expansion of the role of the nurse in primary care. We used as our slogan the words of Halfdan Mahler, the Director General of the WHO: 'If the millions of nurses in a thousand different places articulate the same ideas and convictions about primary health care, and come together as one force, then they could act as a powerhouse for change. I believe that such a change is coming, and that nurses around the globe, whose work touches us intimately, will greatly help to bring it about.'

One problem in the UK was the fragmentation of community services caused by over-specialisation. In the RCN there were 14 Forums representing the different kinds of community nurses by 1990. This was clearly unsustainable, and in November 1990 the Council set up a taskforce on community nursing, which I chaired. There was an internal and an external agenda. My experience has always been that the best way to get people to work together as a team is to get them to work together on a task. The purpose of the taskforce was therefore 'to enable all of the many membership groups within the RCN who are concerned with nursing in the community to work together as a cohesive force to develop, promote, and achieve a clear strategy for community health nursing through the 1990s'. In July 1991 we held a 2-day workshop for representatives of all the relevant membership groups, plus guests from other relevant organisations and experts from other fields – social policy, general practice, health service management and organisations representing consumers and carers. Their work and the results of a mapping exercise to identify needs and problems were distilled into a draft document that was widely circulated and modified by incorporating written submissions from all participants. The revised document was discussed and further modified by a conference of all the relevant interest groups (the consensus conference), which agreed the final version and formally committed itself (and the organisations the participants represented) to it. Two documents were published, both using the title *Powerhouse for Change: a Full Report of the Work*, and a shorter *Manifesto for Community Health Nursing for the 1990s*. The manifesto summarised the values and beliefs that direct community nursing, set out the commitment of community health nurses to accept their identified responsibilities, and strategies for action by community health nurses themselves, health service managers, and government and other health policy makers.

The Clinical Standards Advisory Group

One important committee on which I represented the RCN was the Clinical Standards Advisory Group (CSAG), which was established by the government in 1991 in response to the concerns expressed by the medical profession that reforms then being introduced into the NHS (specifically the 'purchase–provider split') would threaten clinical standards. Secretary of State for Health Kenneth Clarke agreed to establish the CSAG to define clinical standards within the NHS. It included representatives of all the Royal Colleges and was offered a large budget.

Initially the doctors were sceptical. The CSAG first meeting was full of wrangles about how it might work and the proposal was almost rejected; it was the large budget that saved the day. Not for the first time were 'mouths stuffed with gold'. Kenneth Clarke denied that the reforms were introducing a market into health care and stormed out of the meeting, chased by a dozen of the waiting press, shouting: 'Market, what market?'

The way of working was for a small group of CSAG members, accompanied by co-opted experts and research and administrative support, to visit health districts to talk with the new purchasers and providers. In all our studies we found that the new purchasers had little knowledge of what they were purchasing and it was the providers who were specifying the contract, usually based on their current services. In all, 22 studies were completed before the CSAG was replaced by the Commission for Health Improvement 9 years later.

As a member of the CSAG, I took part in several studies. I led the team and wrote much of the report on *Community Health Care for Elderly People.* We used the care of people discharged from hospital after treatment for fractured femur as a tracer condition for identifying the range, level, and quality of community health services for older people. Our report identified the same deficiencies as others, notably the report of the RCN's own research unit. We found poor coordination of discharge plans, lack of interagency collaboration, lack of attention to the rehabilitation needs of older people, and unacceptable variations in service provision according to where people lived and the kind of accommodation they occupied. Primary care teams were feeling the impact of shorter lengths of stay in secondary care, with unacceptable care deficiencies on discharge because of limited health and social care budgets. The rhetoric of 'the money following the patient' was exposed as hollow: older people with increasingly acute needs were being cared for in community settings without a corresponding increase in resources. We called for national standards for care, national eligibility criteria, local rehabilitation services, and a separation in payments between 'health' costs and 'bed and board'. The government's response, published within the Community Health Care report, simply repeated calls for greater collaboration between health and social care services, rather than recognising the need for their integration. We found that no health district was able to make a satisfactory distinction between the two. An editorial on the report in the *British Medical Journal* noted: 'The divide between health and social care needs has enabled health care consistently to evade its responsibility for the continuing care of older people. [...] It seems to be easier to continue with local bickering about who should pay for care rather than take the risk of implementing a national standards framework and costing mechanism.' Our Community Health Care report was instrumental in achieving the establishment of the Royal Commission on Long Term Care a year later, but the same problems persist to this day.

The 75th jubilee

It was the RCN's 75th jubilee year in 1991 and we took 'The value of nursing: to prove, if proof be needed, that nurses make a difference' as our anniversary theme. We produced a 15-minute video about nursing past and present, a magazine supplement about our work, and a booklet of stories contributed by members sharing what is special about nursing through events and incidents in their own clinical practice. As RCN President, I wrote the foreword to both the booklet and supplement.

The year was a round of celebrations. We had a grand birthday party, at which I cut a huge birthday cake. One personal thrill was a kiss from 'Charlie Fairweather' when the team from the TV programme *Casualty* visited Headquarters! There were royal visits and a reception at the House of Commons. During the summer, the Kent and Canterbury Branch held a fête during which I was invited to ascend in a hot air balloon. I was terrified, although I dared not show it, and was greatly relieved to arrive back on terra firma. In addition to these activities, in October there was a service of thanksgiving at Westminster Abbey, at which I read as the second lesson – not a biblical piece, but Gretta Styles' declaration of belief in the nature and purpose of nursing.

Cutting the Jubilee cake

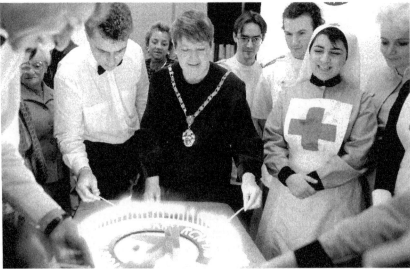

International work

One of the President's roles is to lead the RCN's international work, which was in any case one of my particular interests. As President I chaired the International Committee, whose membership we extended to members with international experience and expertise. For the first time we began to celebrate and popularise International Nurses Day, which is Florence Nightingale's birthday, and that has continued ever since.

Europe

At European level I represented the UK on the EU Advisory Committee on Training in Nursing (ACTN), building on the enormous earlier work of Dame Sheila Quinn in securing the directives that specified the minimum standards required for the recognition of professional qualifications to enable the free movement of (nursing) labour across Europe. The ACTN's remit was to consider basic (pre-registration) general nurse training across the European Union. It was a large committee working in several different languages with simultaneous translation. The ACTN met twice a year in Brussels, and also had two working parties consisting of one representative from each country who met on occasions additional to the plenary sessions. One working party considered the Commission's own interest in the Simplified Legislation in the Internal Market (SLIM) project. It consisted of one representative from each of the seven relevant professions (doctors, nurses, veterinary surgeons, dental practitioners, midwives, architects and pharmacists), and I was appointed to represent nursing. Its brief was to simplify lists of diplomas eligible for automatic recognition, and also to examine whether to transfer the professions concerned to the general system. I learned a great deal about nursing and nursing education across Europe and developed a network of friends who assisted me in other ways, for example in the international programme I was introducing in my 'day job' at Middlesex University. I also learned a great deal about how the EU and Brussels bureaucracy worked, and about working in a variety of languages and cultures. Achieving consensus was not easy.

The International Classification of Nursing Practice

I continued to work with the ICN at several levels. I served on the Professional Services Committee, and worked with Margretta (Gretta) Styles and Norma Lang on the International Classification of Nursing Practice project. This was the work that led me into the field of nursing informatics. It began in 1990 following the acceptance of a motion at the 1989 Council of National Representatives in Seoul, which asked member associations 'to become involved in developing classification systems for nursing care, nursing information management systems, and nursing data sets, in order to provide tools that nurses in all countries can use to describe nursing and its contributions to health'. The aim was to develop a standardised language to describe what nurses do (nursing interventions), for what sort of problems (nursing diagnoses), with what results (nursing outcomes), that could be used to make nursing 'visible' in documentation and information systems. This would enable nursing's contribution to be better recognised, and could create an international database that could be used for comparative research and identification of best practice.

Norma and I were appointed as consultants, working under the guidance of Gretta, Chair of the Professional Services Committee. Having already been involved in trying to describe the work of health visitors in my own research, I was at first somewhat sceptical. Over a drink after our first day's work in Geneva, I asked: 'What are we doing this for?' Norma's casual response: 'If you can't name it you can't control it, finance it, teach it, research it, or put it into public policy' is quoted all around the world and has become the mantra of all those who work in this field. We used it in our initial publication about the project and I often say that if I had a dollar for every time it has been cited or quoted I would now be a millionaire!

The ICNP workshop in Taiwan

ADVISORY MEETING ON ICNP
HOSTED BY ICN/NAROC

This explanation formed the basis for what, over 25 years, has become a worldwide project: the International Classification for Nursing Practice (ICNP). In 1992 we met, again in Geneva, with a panel of nurses from six countries (Chile, Israel, Jamaica, Japan, Kenya and Nepal) to discuss the feasibility and applicability of the work at a global level, and we held further workshops in Mexico in 1994 and in Taiwan in 1995.

In 1993 the first draft of the ICNP was published, consisting of an amalgam of all the terms contained in the then recognised standardised nursing languages; it included as an appendix a review I wrote of the newly-published WHO *International Classification of Diseases* 10th edition (ICD 10), which confirmed the need for a specialist nursing terminology. Norma obtained a large grant from the Kellogg Foundation for expansion in developing countries; and Randi Mortensen, from Denmark, obtained EU funding that enabled translation and testing across Europe. Further drafts followed, until by the end of the decade it became clear that the project needed much more technical expertise than the original developers possessed. In response, the project was restructured to include people from several countries who were experts in the new science of classification, terminology development and the rapidly-developing field of health informatics.

My USA 'reference group'
Gretta and Norma became my close friends and mentors. I stayed at their homes in Milwaukee, Philadelphia, and Florida, where they gave me opportunities to learn about nursing and nursing education in the USA, and I liked what I saw. USA nursing was (and still is) unfairly criticised for being 'all theory and no practice'; I found it more knowledge-based than UK nursing but no less compassionate or skilled. There was no question about the students' 'student status': when groups of students went to the clinical areas they were accompanied by a nurse teacher, who supervised their practice. One interesting initiative at the University of Wisconsin Milwaukee (Norma's first school) was that the School had an agreement with a social housing organisation to provide primary health care services to the residents using nurse practitioners. In addition to the provision of health care, the service provided clinical placements for the students and was also the base for research, including a project to develop a computerised documentation system that used standardised language and retrospective analysis of the database to monitor quality. It was this that I later used as the basis for my work on nursing documentation at Swansea University.

My international work also brought me into contact with the leaders of the American Nurses Association, including Beverly Malone, later to become the RCN's General Secretary, and I was invited to their annual conventions. At one convention I was privileged to meet Hillary Clinton, who came to promote the Clinton Health Care Plan: in such an audience she was speaking to the converted and she received a standing ovation. On another occasion the excitement was outside the conference hall. Having attended all the sessions during the week, I decided that I would spend my last day relaxing by the pool before catching the plane home during the evening. In the middle of the night, however, I was woken by the crash of a carafe of water falling off a table; my 15th floor room was rocking, and I realised I was in the middle of an earthquake. I quickly threw on some clothes, grabbed my bag containing my passport and money, and proceeded to climb down the fire escape – quite the opposite of what I should have done, which was to stay put in my earthquake-proofed room. It was several hours before things returned to normal, so I never got my relaxing day by the pool.

The Romania project

In December 1989, following the downfall of the Ceauşescu regime, the world was shocked by the TV images emerging from Romania of children suffering from AIDS who were incarcerated in Romanian orphanages and hospitals. Among RCN members, as among the rest of the population, there was a huge wave of sympathy, and groups began to form to go to Romania to help. The *Nursing Standard*, led by its Editor, Norah Casey, started a campaign, and we decided to collaborate wherever we could through what became 'the President's Romania project'. Several RCN activists led projects in other parts of the country, but my own activity was focused on the Colentina Hospital, the large infectious diseases hospital in Bucharest where a small British charity called Health Aid UK was working under the inspirational leadership of Anne McNicholas.

Health Aid UK had two main aims: offering themselves and the service they were able to deliver as a role model, and education. In particular, they were trying to develop training for Romanian workers in the hospital. My specific task on my first visit was to cut the ribbon across the door of the little Portakabin that they had placed in the Hospital's grounds to act as the new School of Nursing. The banner above the door proudly bore the legend 'Escuela de Nursing', and the textbook on which the curriculum was built – which was almost their only teaching resource – was Virginia Henderson's little booklet *Basic Principles of Nursing Care*.

During that first visit, I could hardly believe what I saw in the children's wards. There were rows of cots in which children either just lay staring at the ceiling or rocked silently. Some had arms or legs bound to the cot bars 'to keep them safe and stop them falling out'. The stench indicated that nappies were changed infrequently. Babies had crusts around their mouths caused by the practice of leaving them lying down unattended during bottle feeding; for older babies who should have been weaned to solid food, the top of the teat was cut off to enable thickened feeds to be given. The Medical Director, who was pathetically frank in his criticisms of the hospital, showed me around the rest of the hospital. The hospital had been built on the 'villa' principle popular during the 19th century for psychiatric hospitals, in which detached villas were located away from the main building. The design would have been very appropriate as a method of infection control but was not used appropriately. Each villa consisted of one large room into which were crammed some 20 beds so close together that they were almost touching, with a single room at each end. In one villa I visited, the patients were women suffering from tuberculosis; they sat listlessly on their beds just staring into space. In one of the single rooms was a young girl dying of septicaemia as the result of an illegal and botched abortion; in the other was a young man who constantly screamed with pain from meningitis caused by AIDS. In the middle of the ward was a small table and chair at which sat a 'nurse' who was filling in charts. She described herself as a 'medical assistant' and explained that her job consisted of giving the patients injections, dispensing medications (mostly by injection), and keeping the charts up to date for the doctors. She seemed to be quite unaware of the patients, even the screams of the young man. What I found most disturbing was not so much the conditions in which health care was being delivered, but the discovery that the people working in the hospital seemed to have no concept of 'care' or of nursing as we know it. There was not even a word for 'nursing' in the Romanian language. The medical assistants, who were the nearest equivalent health workers to nurses, were proud of their technical skills in, for example, injections and venepuncture, but they did not see the care of the people they carried out these procedures on as any part of their role, and were scornful of our concept of nursing. The hardships of the Ceauşescu period seemed to have drained people, including the hospital workers, of their capacity to care.

Nursing had not always been this way in Romania. Romania had a proud tradition of nursing based on a sound educational programme that had been abolished in favour of the Soviet model. The Romanian Nursing Association

157

(Associatia De Nursing Din Romania) had joined ICN in 1937, but was forced underground during the Ceauşescu regime. The RCN's particular contribution was to work with the Associatia to help it to develop as an educational and organisational resource for its members and to facilitate its re-entry to membership of the ICN. We helped the Associatia to negotiate with the government to achieve professional regulation, and to develop a curriculum for basic nursing education – in the face of opposition from the medical profession, the medical assistants' trade union, and corrupt government officials. I worked in particular with the President of the Associatia, Gabriela Boçek, who was old enough to remember what nursing had been like before the Ceauşescu regime. Somehow she had kept the flame alive in the face of the most terrible circumstances. Sadly Gabriela died of breast cancer a few years later, but I was proud to be present when in 1997 she was made an Honorary Fellow of the RCN and I treasure the little silver medal she gave me on behalf of the Associatia.

Life after my presidency

After my term of office as President ended in 1994, when my role reverted to that of 'ordinary member', people warned me that I would feel a tremendous sense of bereavement. It did not happen: I was far too busy with other aspects of my work. For a few years I did keep a low profile in the RCN. I continued to attend Congress and AGMs, and I continued most of my international activities, especially the work on the ICNP.

Investiture as DBE

Being invested as a Dame Commander of the Order of the British Empire in 1995 undoubtedly marked the peak of my career. I knew that it was not uncommon for presidents of Royal Colleges (both medical and nursing) to receive a Queen's honour on retiring from office, so in one sense perhaps I should not have been so surprised. My father, who had been awarded an OBE a generation earlier in recognition of his contribution to the post-war redevelopment of Wales, was somewhat sceptical about such things, rudely describing his own award as 'Other Buggers Efforts' – although he was of course very proud underneath! But I was stunned by the proposal to make me a Dame!

The great day was organised like a military operation. Christine Hancock had generously provided a chauffeur-driven limousine to take us to the Palace. Roger and both children accompanied me. All the ladies wore hats and gloves. My daughter Gillian was resplendent in a hat that looked like a wedding cake. I looked and felt ridiculous in my new outfit; it was the first time in years that I had worn a skirt rather than trousers. The men were in morning dress or military uniforms covered in gold braid. We felt like royalty as we swept up the Mall and the gates opened before us. Now that Buckingham Palace has been opened to the public some of the mystique has disappeared. Despite this, no-one could fail to be impressed by the beautiful red and gold decor of the ballroom (where the investiture takes place), or the pictures on the walls in the grand corridor. The feature that I especially remember, however, is the lavatory: it was a wooden bench with a hole in it, just like the privy my grandma had in her back garden, except that this one was made of the most beautiful polished mahogany.

Once in, we were colour-coded into the 'sheep and the goats': while the guests and the 'lower orders' went in one direction, I was wafted to the Green Room for a more private briefing with the four gentlemen who were being knighted. The master-at-arms spent 20 minutes demonstrating how the new knights should kneel in front of the Zimmer-like frame for the Queen to touch their shoulders with the sword. When I cheekily asked if he would show me how to curtsey, he demurred. Regretting my faux pas, I murmured that perhaps I could just copy the person in front of me. In response to this, he drew himself up over his gold braid and said: 'Dame June, you are the most senior person today. You will be first!'

At Buckingham Palace for June's DBE investiture

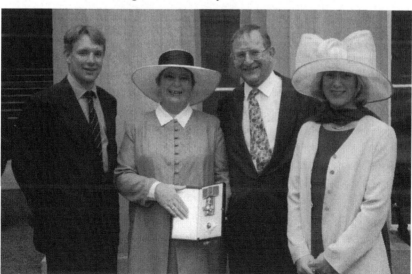

We had to wait in a long line while we were checked and re-checked until our turn came. When our name was called we walked forward to a place marked on the carpet and turned to face the Queen. In my role as RCN President I had met the Queen and other members of the royal family before. I never fail to admire the professionalism with which they carry out their duties. When it was my turn, the Queen took the insignia medal from the equerry beside her and fastened it onto the hook that had previously been pinned to my coat. She was extraordinarily well briefed and seemed to know all about me and about what I did. It was at the time when the Queen Mother had just been in hospital for a hip replacement, so I said I hoped she was being well looked after and we spoke for several minutes. After receiving my medal, I had to take two steps backwards, turn to the right, and walk out. The equerry removed the insignia, put it into a little box and gave it back to me. And that was it. It was all over. Out into the rain, without even a cup of tea! However cynical I may seem about other aspects of the process, the words 'Professor Dame June Clark: for services to nursing' still make the goose pimples rise on the back of my neck: it was a magical moment. After the ceremony we went back to RCN headquarters for a party, and then home in our chauffeur-driven car for a family celebration. It was a day to be remembered.

I rarely use the title Dame, except on formal occasions and in the formal records of meetings (especially of meetings dominated by titled men!). And I hate it when people are deferential because of it. Some months after my investiture I went to Brazil to speak at a conference alongside Marjorie Gordon and Sue Bakken, doyens of standardised nursing languages in the USA. Our hostess was very worried about how to introduce me. Sue, who has a wonderfully dry sense of humour, said: 'No problem! There are three of us: two Americans and a Brit. You just introduce us as two broads and a dame!' In the RCN in particular I insist on being referred to as June and not Dame June. I am proud of the award, however, most especially because I see it as an honour not just for me, but for nursing.

The Virginia Henderson Memorial Lecture

In 1997 the ICN Congress was held in Vancouver, Canada. I had planned to go with my longstanding friend Jean Cubbin, but when I was appointed to my new post at Swansea University I felt I could not ask for leave so soon. In any case, I was not sure that I could afford it – the cost of registration, travel, and accommodation was considerable. Then came an invitation I simply could not refuse. Following the death of Virginia Henderson, whom many would regard as the '20th century Florence Nightingale', the ICN decided to commemorate her life and work with a Virginia Henderson Memorial Lecture to be given at each future ICN congress. I was invited to give the inaugural lecture on the theme of 'The unique function of the nurse' – Henderson's definition of nursing that is recognised and still used by nurses all over the word. I was quite overwhelmed: I knew that they could have chosen any nurse from anywhere in the world.

The problem was that I was so overwhelmed that I was like a rabbit paralysed in the headlights of an oncoming car. I had 3 months to prepare the lecture, and the theme could not have been nearer to my heart, but somehow it just would not 'come' and I was still struggling with it when I arrived in Vancouver. It was a good job that Jean accompanied me. Every morning until the great day she ensured that I got out of bed at 7am, dropped me into the swimming pool for half an hour, forced me to eat breakfast, then sat me in front of my computer to write. By the day before the lecture was due the translators were agitating for the script and the audiovisual technicians wanted my slides, and I could provide neither. I gave the translators the unfinished draft, and the technicians a few generic slides that I thought I could fit in somewhere. On the morning of the lecture Jean put her foot down. 'That's it,' she said. 'You just have to do it.'

So I did. I was so nervous that I completely forgot to use the slides. Fortunately there was a background slide of Virginia Henderson herself, which stayed on screen throughout. When I finished there was absolute silence in the hall for what seemed like an eternity but was probably only a few seconds. Then there was a great roar and 3000 people were on their feet, clapping and stamping. During my presidency and on other occasions I have received many standing ovations, but never one like this. Fortunately the next agenda item was coffee, so, somewhat dazed, I made my way through the crowd towards the coffee point. I never got there because so many people wanted to congratulate me. What seemed strange to me is that I thought then, and I still believe, that nothing that I said was new, that what I said was no more than the daily stock in trade of every nurse in every country of the world. It was a nurse from China, speaking in rather broken English, who pointed out that it was exactly this that had impressed her, and this was the reason people had reacted in the way they did. The speech was translated into several languages and published in several nursing journals in other countries in addition to the ICN's *International Nursing Review*. Over the following year I was asked to repeat it at conferences in Switzerland, Ireland, Finland and Denmark.

161

Defining Nursing

I undertook just one more major piece of work for the RCN. As a result of my work with Norma and Gretta, I was introduced to a document first published by the American Nurses Association in 1980 called *Nursing: A Social Policy Statement*; Norma had led the working party that developed it. All of a sudden, many of the issues about the nature and purpose of nursing that I had wrestled with for years fell into place. The document defines the nature and scope of the practice of nursing, and sets it in its social context, sets out its values, and distinguishes the different types and levels of nursing practice. Updated in 1995, 2003 and 2010, it still forms the bedrock of all policy development in the American Nurses Association.

When I read the American Nurses Association statement, I realised that something like this was desperately needed for British nursing, which was – and still is – struggling with its own identity. In the UK several developments were increasing the need to develop a more explicit description of the service nurses can offer, and to differentiate the particular contribution of nursing within the framework of the multidisciplinary health care team. Nurses were extending their roles in many ways. There were also external drivers: for example, cost containment measures coupled with a shortage of registered nurses were leading to skill-mix exercises in which work formerly undertaken by registered nurses was transferred to other staff. Research in the early 80s was beginning to show that the proportion of registered nurses in the workforce affects patient outcomes, such as speed of recovery, incidence of complications, and even mortality – although it did not explain why. At the same time, pressures on the availability of doctors meant that nurses were taking on some of their work. Research, for example on the work of nurse practitioners, was showing that nurses can undertake a great deal of the work previously undertaken by doctors safely and competently and that patients appreciate it. I put the case for publication of a similar document for the UK to Christine Hancock, then General Secretary, who – ever the pragmatist – thought it was far too theoretical for British nursing.

Almost a decade went by until, following the government's rejection of the recommendations of the Royal Commission on Long Term Care, the Health and Social Care Act 2001 drew a distinction between nursing care that would be funded by the NHS and free of charge to the user at the point of delivery, and 'personal care', which would be provided through local authority social services departments and therefore paid for by the patient subject to means testing. There is nothing more practical than having to pay for something. When I gave evidence to the newly-established Welsh Assembly about the Royal Commission's report, one Assembly member immediately commented: 'So it all depends on your definition of nursing.' She then turned to the civil servants who were present and asked: 'Is this a devolved responsibility?' Before they could reply, I quickly interrupted: 'Well the definition of nursing is a matter for the profession'. And then, lying through my teeth: 'I'm sure the Royal College of Nursing can provide you with one.' Tina Donnelly, the Director of RCN Wales, was sitting in the public gallery, and she and I worked together to provide the promised statement by the end of the week. Sadly HQ did not move quickly enough, and in the absence of any professional definition the legislative definition of nursing care – which still stands – was formulated by civil servants as: '… any services provided by a registered nurse and involving – (a) the provision of care, or (b) the planning, supervision or delegation of the provision of care, other than any services which, having regard to their nature and the circumstances in which they are provided, do not need to be provided by a registered nurse.' This begs the question of what services need to be provided by a registered nurse, and has caused professional and legal wrangling ever since.

Meanwhile, Beverly Malone had succeeded Christine as General Secretary. As a former president of the American Nurses Association, she fully understood the significance of *Nursing: A Social Policy Statement*. On her advice, Council agreed to establish a taskforce, and I was named project leader, assisted by a steering group that included the immediate past president (Sylvia Denton), three members of Council (Jackie Burns, Diane Rawstorne, and Eirlys Warrington) and staff support including the Executive Director for Nursing (Alison Kitson). We undertook an extensive literature search, surveyed national nurses associations around the world to find out what definitions were currently used (by far the most common were Henderson's definition of 'the unique function of the nurse' and the definition given in *Nursing: A Social Policy Statement*), and carried out a 'values clarification exercise' using the tool developed by Alison Kitson and Kim Manley. The values clarification exercise produced some worrying results that confirmed the need for our work: nurses were able to describe the purpose of nursing, usually using the concepts in Henderson's definition, but were unable to articulate how they achieved it or the specific knowledge base on which their practice was built. Our first draft was circulated to all membership groups and their comments were incorporated. This made the definition longer than we had hoped because every nursing specialty wanted their particular contribution specified, but we were helped by a clever graphics designer who was able to express what we wanted as a simple diagram showing a core surrounded by a periphery of six defining characteristics. A whole day at RCN Congress was devoted to discussion of the final document, which was approved by Council and published in 2003 with the title *Defining Nursing*. We wrote:

'*The RCN expects that nurses will be able to use this document to:*

- *Describe nursing to people who do not understand it*
- *Clarify their role in the multidisciplinary health care team*
- *Influence the policy agenda at local and national level*
- *Develop educational curricula*
- *Identify areas where research is needed to strengthen the knowledge base of nursing*
- *Inform decisions about whether and how nursing work should be delegated to other personnel*
- *Support negotiations at local and national level on issues such as nurse staffing, skill mix and nurses' pay.'*

Sadly, *Defining Nursing* failed to achieve its potential. It has rarely been used in subsequent policy development. To this day I do not understand why. Meanwhile the confusion over nursing roles and the tension between professional nursing and the scope of practice of the support worker continues.

Defining Nursing

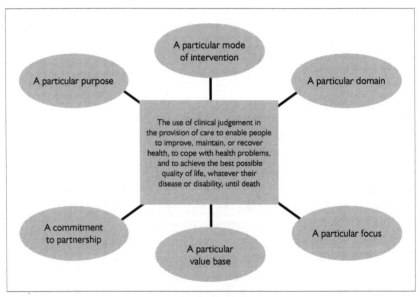

PART 4: THE ROYAL COLLEGE OF NURSING: THE ENDING OF THE AFFAIR

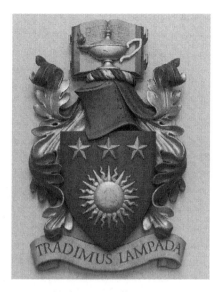

The RCN coat of arms, granted by the College of Heralds in 1946.*

CHAPTER 11: DECLINE AND FALL

When Roger described me as 'married to the RCN' he spoke the truth. For more than 40 years, beginning when I was still a student nurse, I was deeply involved with the RCN. I served as Branch Secretary, Branch Chair, and Branch PR Officer, Council member, Chair of RRB, Deputy President, and finally President. I am sure that my investiture as Dame was also a recognition of my work in the RCN. The RCN was 'in my blood', and I was proud of my contribution.

As the 20th century gave way to the 21st, however, there was a dramatic change in the orientation and culture of the RCN that challenged my deepest values about what a membership organisation should be, and

---

*The RCN coat of arms bears the motto *Tradimus Lampada*, meaning 'we hand on the torch'. The College was the first organisation of women to receive a shield rather than a lozenge shape to emblazon its arms, paying tribute to the wartime service of the College and its members. The shield shows the sun and stars denoting the day and night service that nurses provide. This is surmounted by the open book of learning and a Roman oil lamp which is the authorized heraldic symbol of nursing, as decided by the College of Heralds.

167

culminated in my withdrawal from RCN activities for nearly 7 years. It was like the ending of a love affair. It broke my heart.

Way back in 1977, when conflict between the RCN and the TUC-affiliated trade unions was at its height, I wrote an article in the *Nursing Mirror* entitled 'Why I chose the RCN'. I argued that the interaction between the RCN's multiple functions was its greatest strength. I argued that in labour relations the key difference between the RCN and other trade unions was a difference between ends and means: that whereas for other trade unions the protection of members' interests was an end in itself, for the RCN this was merely a proper means of achieving the primary end of improving patient care. This is why the RCN's first objective as set out in its charter – 'To promote the science and art of nursing and the education and training in the profession of nursing' – was so important. I argued the importance of the organisation being composed exclusively of nurses and governed by nurses, because only nurses have the specialist expertise, values, and understanding that enables them to represent nurses' views.

In the 1970s almost all the RCN staff (other than the secretaries) were nurses, so whatever the additional skill set they used in their RCN job – whether in labour relations, public relations, policy development, etc – they knew what it felt like to be a nurse because they had been there and done it. Nowadays the majority of RCN staff members are not nurses, representation for members may be provided by people who are not nurses, and there have even been moves to remove the requirement that the General Secretary should be a nurse. By 2013, out of 940 employed staff, only 62 were in the Nursing Department – fewer than in RCN Publishing (86) or RCN Direct (the RCN telephone helpline), which had 90.

In 2000 the RCN opened its membership to health care assistants and associate practitioners. This was a move no doubt right for a trade union wanting to become the biggest health services union, but entirely wrong, in my view, for a professional association. Sadly, therefore, I question whether the RCN is still a professional association because the promotion of the science and art of nursing is no longer its first objective, and the inclusion of other health workers in its membership means that it is just a trade union for health workers like any of its competitors.

It is only with hindsight that I can see what was happening and can now understand why the love affair ended. To quote Father Oscar Romero: 'There are many things that can only be seen through eyes that have cried.' In the months that followed I cried plenty.

Still a professional association?

The shift in focus towards the RCN's trade union function was made explicit in the changes to the RCN charter in 2010, as a result of which the RCN ceased to be a charity. A Foundation was established as a means of managing charitable income, but nothing replaced the professional functions previously undertaken by the Forums.

I became concerned about this trend as early as the mid 1990s. When the annual report for 1995/6 was published, I wrote to the *Nursing Standard* to complain. I complained that the first four of its eleven pages were about NHS pay and conditions of service followed by two pages about retirements, appointments, and the external achievements of individual members; there were two pages about the work of the External Affairs Department. There was not a word about the science and art of nursing, not a word about nursing education, not a word about policy for nursing, nursing practice, about preparing nurses for the rapid changes in healthcare. I suggested that the RCN had lost its way, that it had forgotten that it was a Royal College, that it had become just – as its documents constantly proclaimed –'the world's largest (professional) union of nurses'.

Christine Hancock, then General Secretary, was furious. Pat Hughes, Chair of Council, took us both out to dinner to talk through the issue. Balance was restored in the next few annual reports, and over the next few years the RCN held an Autumn Conference that combined the conferment of Fellowships, a professional conference, a presidential address and the AGM. The idea was to have two major meetings in each year: a political meeting (Congress) in the spring; and a professional meeting (to include the AGM) in the autumn. The autumn meeting was intended to showcase the RCN as a professional association but from 2007 the practice was dropped, and from 2014 the AGM was subsumed within Congress. The resultant change in the composition of the voting attendance, with an increase in numbers but a bias in favour of activists, is significant.

There are several other indicators of this shift in focus. One is the presentation of the College's purposes and priorities in documents such as annual reports. The first purpose of the RCN as stated in its charter is: 'To promote the science and art of nursing and education and training in the profession of nursing.' This purpose, however, has been gradually superseded by the current mission statement: 'The RCN represents nurses and nursing, promotes excellence in practice, and shapes health policies.' In annual reports and in the 'About Us' page of the website, the first purpose as set out in the charter is now relegated to the second bullet point under the fourth sub-heading of the mission statement.

The loss of educational and research functions

Another indicator is what has happened to the educational and research functions that had made the RCN the recognised leading source of expert knowledge and expertise about professional nursing. The charter states: 'There shall be within the College an educational institution for the purposes of furthering the better education of the nursing profession. The governance and structure of the Institute shall be set out in Regulations.'

As early as 1918 the (then) College of Nursing established an Education Department and over the years came to be seen as the main source of expertise about nursing education. It led policy development and was a major provider of post-registration education (pre-registration was undertaken by hospital-based schools of nursing), especially at more senior levels such as nurse teachers and nurse managers. Its international management programme attracted nurses from all over the world. By 1971, when the Education Department became the Institute for Advanced Nursing Education, it was providing a wide range of degree and diploma programmes in association with several universities and from five centres around the country: London, Birmingham, Edinburgh, Belfast, and Cardiff. It was pioneering courses in new fields, such as AIDS nursing and (later) nurse practitioners in primary care, and validating courses run by other organisations. As nursing education developed in the universities, its role and organisational structure changed but its reputation was maintained and enhanced.

The RCN also took a lead in the development of nursing research. In the 1960s it had undertaken the first major nursing research project on the quality of nursing care. Throughout the 70s and 80s it published a series of research monographs, including three of mine. In 1982 it established the Daphne Heald Research Unit (named in honour of Lady Daphne Heald who had been a Vice-President of the College and for more than 20 years Chair of its Appeals Committee). I chaired the committee that established it, and the Council's Research Committee for several years. In 1995 the Daphne Heald Research Unit merged with the Institute of Advanced Nursing Education to form the RCN Institute. The biennial review of the RCN Institute for 1998–2000 lists 186 members of full-time and associated staff, and records seven pages of publications, eight pages of conference presentations, and two pages of funding grants during the period covered. At that time no one could doubt the RCN's key role in 'promoting the science and art of nursing'. From the turn of the century, however, the RCN's research and educational activity gradually declined, and in 2007, as part of an internal management re-organisation, the RCN Institute disappeared from the organisational structure; its Director left and was not replaced. Many members now question whether the RCN still complies with its charter.

Changes in the RCN management structure

In 2007, following the appointment of Peter Carter as the incoming General Secretary, the Executive Team was changed to comprise the Directors of Governance Support, Human Resources, Legal Services, Finance and Corporate Services, and Communications, the Directors of the four countries that make up the UK, and the Director of Nursing and Service Delivery. The post of Director of Nursing disappeared, and since then there has been no recognisable lead for the professional side of the College. The Director of Nursing at that time was Alison Kitson, and her responsibilities had included leading the RCN Institute. She had been recognised nationally and internationally as a leader in the development of 'the science and art of nursing'. Even more important, however, was her visibility and profile as the lead for the professional side of the RCN. I believe that the loss of the post of Director of Nursing was hugely significant.

I am not the only one to be concerned about this shift away from professional issues; it is repeatedly raised by those members who joined the RCN because it was a professional association (although it has to be recognised that many members join only for the protection it provides on employment matters). In 2013, an editorial in the *British Journal of Nursing* asked: 'Has the RCN lost its way? Members may struggle to obtain advice and support on professional and clinical issues. There may be other organisations that support the learning, knowledge and professional development of nurses with a commitment to making a difference to health, but the RCN may no longer be one of them.'

The tensions between multiple purposes

There have always been tensions between the multiple and sometimes conflicting purposes and functions of the RCN. The original purposes for which the RCN was founded were educational and professional, although from the very beginning the RCN was in the forefront of battles to improve the pay and conditions of nurses. In 1977 the RCN registered as a trade union under the Trade Union and Labour Relations Act, which gave it the same rights and obligations as other trade unions but allowed it to retain its charitable status. I have always supported the RCN's trade union functions but professionalism has always been my driver, and I saw the RCN as the vehicle through which it could be achieved and maintained.

The 2006 Charities Act challenged the RCN's charitable status and forced a review of its governance arrangements. This was the opportunity to do what nursing associations in some other countries have done: to develop two organisations, one a trade union and the other a professional association, which would work together in partnership. Sweden, for example, has the Swedish Society of Nursing (Svensk Sjuksköterskeförening), which is 'the professional organisation for nurses and represents the profession's areas of expertise with a view to promoting research, education and development and quality development in nursing', and the Swedish Association of Health Professionals (Vårdförbundet), which is the trade union that represents nurses, midwives and radiographers. The two organisations work closely together. Switzerland has a similar arrangement. In the UK the Health Visitors' Association (now part of the Unite trade union) has established a Health Visiting Institute.

In the various consultation and information documents issued by RCN Council, there was no mention of alternative models and it was never explained why this option was chosen in preference to others: all meetings and papers were classed as 'confidential', and 'consultation' documents merely promoted the proposals that were being made and urged members to vote for them. The changes, combined with those made by the governance review, have, in my view, greatly inhibited the role of the RCN as a member-led professional organisation.

The model that the RCN chose to follow was to create the RCN Foundation, a charity and a private company limited by guarantee whose function is to raise and dispense funds. I am not opposed to the creation of the Foundation, but clearly it does not serve the same function as a professional organisation. It is not a membership organisation; it is a private company that is governed and controlled entirely by independent trustees/directors.

The changes have left a gap. As England's (then) Chief Nursing Officer, Dame Christine Beasley, remarked in the evidence she presented at the Mid Staffordshire NHS inquiry in June 2011: 'I do think one of the things we lack is an independent Royal College that can do some of the things that royal colleges of doctors and medicine do.' I agree. Even within the RCN's trade union function there are conflicts. In her autobiography *From SRN to CBE*, Mary Spinks describes her dilemma when, as a senior nurse manager, she had to take disciplinary action against nurses responsible for poor care who were represented and supported by the RCN – of which she too was a member – and which she expected to support her in upholding standards of care. This potential conflict was highlighted by Robert Francis in his report on the Mid Staffordshire NHS Foundation Trust: 'There is an inherent conflict between the professional representative and trade union functions of the RCN which may diminish the authority of its voice on professional issues.' Several of his witnesses agreed. Dame Christine said in evidence that while there were some advantages to combining the union and the professional organisation in the RCN, these were outweighed by the conflict of interest. The current debate over funding nursing education is another example.

Responding to the Francis Report, RCN Chief Executive and General Secretary Peter Carter said the College had 'carefully considered' Francis' suggestion that the organisation should split its functions, but that 'the membership' (in the form of a vote at the 2013 Congress) had voted overwhelmingly against it. Separation of the two functions has been discussed many times, but has always been presented as splitting the organisation, and been rejected mainly in the belief that nurses, who would see membership of a trade union as essential protection, would not be willing to pay for a professional association. I do not see the creation of two separate organisations as splitting the RCN: the trade union could retain all the RCN's present activities (although there might be a fight over the title), while an independent Royal College would, as Dame Christine suggested, function in ways similar to the medical Royal Colleges.

In 2013 there came, what was for me, the final insult: the RCN withdrew from membership of the International Council of Nurses (ICN), the global network of national nursing organisations that the RCN itself had founded more than a century ago. ICN is also the nursing profession's entry gate to other international organisations, such as the World Health Organization, the World Health Assembly and UN agencies. My work within the ICN and attendance at its conferences ever since my student days was hugely influential in developing my views about nursing. That is why I have now established a travel scholarship to enable Welsh nurses to have the same opportunities as I enjoyed. The reason given for the RCN's withdrawal was that the expense of membership did not provide value for money to RCN members. This was a further indicator of narrow trade union priorities and business orientation over any commitment to the profession as a whole or to what an organisation such as the RCN could offer to the profession worldwide.

The governance review

The changes required by the 2006 legislation became part of a wide-ranging governance review that extended to every RCN activity and membership entity. The constitutions, functions, and ways of working of committees, forums, regional boards, and branches were replaced by new rules and regulations. The process was masterminded by a newly-established Governance Support Unit, which rapidly became the most powerful department in the organisation. The Governance Support Officer became a Director and a member of the Executive team.

It was always my habit to go to say hello to new members of staff and to offer my services – jokingly – as the 'memory' of the organisation they were joining. Some time during 2006 I went to see the newly-appointed Governance Support Officer. We chatted amicably for maybe half an hour, during which time she told me about her previous work with the National Trust and other charities. I remember reflecting, as I left, about how their governance arrangements, which must reflect their norms and values, differed from those of a membership organisation such as ours.

I did not see any particular significance in the thought at the time and dismissed it from my mind. It was much later, in a Discussion Zone thread about the RCN's new governance arrangements, that I remembered it and realised its significance for the changes that were being made in the governance of the RCN. My posting on the Discussion Zone to this effect was considered by the General Secretary to be 'offensive' and was swiftly removed. With hindsight it is probably the truest thing I ever said.

The 'norms and values' that I had in mind go to the very heart of the definition of a membership organisation. The 'value' is that a membership organisation belongs to its members; the 'norm' is that this is achieved through membership participation in a bottom-up system of representative democracy – the system by which members elect other members to take decisions on their behalf. Members participate in the activities of the organisation both directly in meetings of various kinds and through their elected representatives. It is this that enables an organisation to describe itself as 'member-led'.

In 2007 this 'participatory governance model' was replaced by what was called a 'downward delegation model'. An organisational chart on the RCN website depicted the new governance model. Arrows showed the downward flow of decisions from the Council, its committees, and the boards to the members in the branches, but there were no upward arrows. The model offered no scope for 'upward participation' by members. Elections were now abandoned; instead, committees were appointed in a formal selection process managed by the governance support unit, so the principles of representation and accountability were lost. Members became 'customers' and a project 'to look at the way the RCN delivers customer services' was started. Within a few years the RCN was transformed. As a letter to me from the General Secretary said 'The RCN has moved on.... It is a different organisation.'

Although Council approved the changes, members were not consulted and certainly did not agree to them. At the time I, and I suspect most other members, did not recognise what was happening. Even if we had, within the new governance model we were powerless to do anything about it.

The 'rationalisation' of the Forums

The biggest, and perhaps the most disastrous, aspect of these changes, however, was the 'rationalisation' of the Forums. Forums had been created to support the specialist interests of members, which the 1973 membership reorganisation had clearly shown the members wanted.

The functions of forums were set out in their Constitution as:

- To provide a focus for members to participate in professional activities
- To provide an expert resource to Council and the membership
- To develop policy and practice related to [forum-specific] nursing, recognising the diversity across the United Kingdom
- To provide the opportunity for RCN members engaged in [forum-specific] nursing to meet together, to network and to increase their knowledge and skills and so enhance their practice
- To encourage all nurses engaged in [forum-specific] nursing to join the RCN.

Some Forums worked better than others, but any review of the RCN's work during the 1980s and 90s demonstrates the enormous contribution they made. I had been an active member of five Forums, served as an elected member of the steering committees of three, and became Chair of the IN Forum. The Forums were the main vehicle for carrying out the RCN's professional work, since it was forum members that constituted the College's professional expertise. As one forum chair wrote: 'It is important to consider that our professional colleagues both in the UK and in Europe absolutely respect the RCN as having influence professionally because of its unique and large scale capacity to seek and include the views of its membership in developing contemporary nursing through influencing policy and action in areas of specialised practice. The RCN is respected even as a global resource because of this very capacity, and its views are sought. If the Forums go... then so does this element of the RCN's portfolio,

175

and this is an irretrievable commodity, because others will take this work and the respect that goes with it. The RCN simply becomes another union.' This is exactly what happened.

The Forums became a victim of their own success. By 2005 it was clear that there were too many forums and there were problems with their management, especially their financial management. The Council had already initiated an internal review called the Professional Development Project 'to modernise and streamline the RCN's professional services to members' and several taskforces were established covering various aspects of the RCN's work. One of these, called the Professional Membership Structure (PMS) project, was directed towards the Forums. In September 2005 a consultation document was circulated outlining the PMS project, stating: 'RCN members will be central to forming this vision', but only a month after the consultation closed and without any further discussion the Council decided that 'existing national Forums become either virtual or local networks'. This proposal was embedded in a package of recommendations proposed to Council by the Professional Development Project Management Board, was not included in the consultation document, and was passed without discussion or consultation with the Forums' chairs.

In a letter to the *Nursing Standard* on 8 March I wrote: 'The Concise Oxford definition of "virtual" is "not physically existing as such, but made by software to appear so" – perhaps unwittingly a very accurate description of Council's intention.... Thus at a single stroke the RCN forums as we know them are abolished.... Forums constitute the professional expertise of the RCN without which the RCN cannot meet the definition of a professional association and becomes just another trade union.'

It was clear to many of us that the proposal that Forums become virtual networks was based on a complete misunderstanding of the purposes and limitations of social networking.

The Information in Nursing Forum (IN Forum) submitted a proposal to establish two virtual networks (one for nurses working in informatics and one for Forum members in Scotland). The proposal was rejected by the Forums Governance Group (FGG) on the grounds that the Cardiac Nurses Network (whose chair was also the chair of the FGG) was being established as a pilot. Two years later the FGG were forced to admit that the Cardiac Nurses Network had not been evaluated and no criteria had been determined to evaluate other virtual Forums.

A Forum Activists' Listserv was started and a website called Voice of Nursing: Save Your Forum established. Council members were lobbied and there were letters to the nursing press, all protesting at the proposals. In the run-up to Congress, a petition was submitted asking Council 'to suspend their decision [that forums become local or virtual networks] until there is evidence that such a change would be feasible.' The petition was ignored. On Sunday, the day before Congress began, the forum chairs met. On Monday we demonstrated outside the Congress hall. On Tuesday the Council hosted a question and answer meeting on the Professional Development Project and PMS. On Wednesday a panel of Council members met with the forum activists and agreed that the forum representation on the Professional Membership Structure Implementation Group (later renamed the Professional Membership Structure Action Group and consisting mainly of Council members and RCN staff) would be increased to six. In June the election for these places was held; there were 29 candidates, and the turnout was 51% – the largest turnout ever recorded in an RCN election.

The campaign continued through to 2008. Forum Chairs' days run by the FGG were used as platforms to tell Forum chairs of what had already been decided; there was never space on the agenda for questions or discussion, and Forum chairs were not invited to contribute items to the agenda. The PMS Action Group established six workgroups to deal in depth with the various aspects of Forums that needed attention. Throughout 2006 and 2007 the workgroups worked; we identified the financial deficiencies that were later exposed by the RCN auditors; we reviewed the Forum Constitution, identified the technological needs, and started work on reducing the number of Forums. We agreed that all existing Forums should be required to re-apply to Council to be formally recognised as Forums, and developed a set of criteria against which the applications would be judged. We estimated that this process would encourage mergers of Forums whose specialist areas overlapped, and substantially reduce the number of forums. All this was done to develop the consensus that we knew would be necessary to persuade the Forum chairs to accept some hard decisions. As Chair of the main workgroup, I prepared endless documents setting out our proposals and the work we had done. All were totally ignored. The functions and ways of working laid down in the Forum Constitution were simply overruled. The Forum Constitution itself 'disappeared'.

Initially, meetings of the Forums were reduced in frequency to two per year, to start no earlier than 11 am and finish by 4 pm, but soon even these meetings were cut. Forum budgets were removed and centralised. All Forum activity had to be approved by the FGG, which was serviced by the Governance Support Unit, which appointed Forum committees. Forum newsletters were reduced from four to one a year and direct communication between Forum members and their committees was prevented by a ruling that members' email addresses could not be made available to Forum officers; all emails had to be filtered through the Governance Support Unit. The ability of the elected Forum steering committees to manage their own affairs was effectively removed.

At the height of the battle, in September 2008, a former member of staff who had worked for several years with forums wrote to the Director of Governance Support, saying that he remained unconvinced that there had been the level of critical thinking and analysis needed to deliver equal and necessary support to the professional arm of the College. He believed that the RCN still underestimated the importance and the power of RCN professional forums. He argued that Forums and specialty specific information still remained an important part of why nurses joined the RCN instead of Unison... Some forums had really exciting and busy plans which covered publications, political lobbying, guideline development, organising professional conferences, running their web communities etc etc.

He said that he supported a reduction in the number of Forums and definitely believed there was scope for merging some groups where there was overlap or similar objectives. However, he said that as a former member of the staff involved he wished to make it clear that the proposed changes were not widely discussed or worked on by the Nursing Department. In fact discussion had been limited to a brief 10-minute exercise on an Awayday sticking a few pieces of paper on the wall with some very early personal thoughts. That was as scientific as it got! He believed that the new operational planning process was cumbersome, time consuming, and in many ways detached from reality, and that having seen the feedback for many of the forum operational plans, he was clear that the reviewers were often unaware of the importance of some of the work streams. Asking Forums to deliver their workload and operational plan in two face to face meetings and a short teleconference was simply not achievable. We are essentially asking them, he suggested, to work with one hand tied behind their back.

Finally, in January 2009 the report of the FGG, which had now taken over the work of the PMS Action Group (which had been abolished), stated: 'there would be no further [Forum] Steering Committee meetings after April 2009. All meetings would be around activity streams. Rather than submit operational plans in 2009–10 Forums will be submitting project bids for specific pieces of work throughout the year. The FGG would approve each of the bids against agreed criteria.'

The Forums were bullied into submission. The RCN Annual Report for 2009–10 noted that the Forums Rationalisation Project was now complete, and that it had been 'very successful'. The Forums as they used to be had gone, and with them a large chunk of the RCN's credibility as a professional association.

The proposed sale of 20 Cavendish Square

In 2006 RCN was in financial difficulties, mainly as a result of a large pensions deficit. The Council's proposed solution to the financial problems was to sell the Headquarters building. Once again, the decision was made in a private session and leaked. When the decision became public at the 2006 AGM a campaign co-ordinating committee was formed; it was chaired by Jane Denton, a well-respected Fellow of the RCN, and included Mamie Bishopp-Schyberg, Gerry Bolger, Dave Dawes, Reynagh Jarrett, Chris McDonnell, Maria Nicholson, Peggy Prior, Jan Rushford, and myself. As with the decision to make Forums virtual entities, we were able to demonstrate that the Council's decision was based on inadequate and inaccurate information. We showed that there were better ways of solving the pension problem, and that it was not feasible, even if it had been desirable, to pursue the sale. We mobilised the provision in the byelaws that Council must call an extraordinary general meeting on a petition of 1000 members. The petition was set up, the requisite number of signatures was obtained, and the Extraordinary General Meeting was scheduled during Congress 2007. It was very well attended and far exceeded the required number of members for a quorum. The meeting voted overwhelmingly to stop the sale and for the new General Secretary, Peter Carter, to prepare and present a financial recovery plan to members at the next AGM. Council decided not to pursue the sale.

The process exposed a number of problems within the organisation. One was the absolute power of Council to act without consultation with members, which perhaps explains some of the problems of the PMS project. Most importantly, events had demonstrated that all was not well in the relationships between Headquarters staff, Council, and ordinary members.

Although he had not yet taken up post, Peter Carter came to the 2006 AGM and heard these debates. I introduced myself, welcomed him, and whispered: 'You are taking over a very dysfunctional organisation.' In the battles that followed he often reminded me of this comment. He had been a member of the RCN but never an activist. He came with the reputation that in his 11 years as Chief Executive of the Central and North West London Mental Health Trust, the Trust had never been in deficit. During his first year in post at the RCN, he turned the organisation around financially, pushed through a revised pension scheme and tightened financial and staff management. For this he deserves credit, perhaps more than he has received. The directorates were reorganised and a new Executive Team was developed; several senior staff 'left'.

Under new management

The new governance structure and the appointment of the new General Secretary were accompanied by the development of a centralised 'command and control' style of management. This played a large part in the breakdown of my own personal relationship with the RCN. The implementation of the changes was the worst example of change management I had ever experienced and it affected me deeply.

Central control soon led to changes to branches, boards and all other parts of the organisation. On the Discussion Zone, one longstanding activist suggested that this review would have a fundamental impact on governance within the organisation and would impact on every member. He said that although he was chair of one of the largest branches in the UK, he had no idea what the proposals were and that this was the case for most members. He pointed out that the plans, which had been going on for nearly 3 years, had happened at closed sessions of the regional and country boards; very few board members had actually discussed these changes at local level and were therefore unable to comment.

Another pointed out that this was the third example of structural proposals made without members' agreement/consultation in about 4 years. She demanded that not only should this proposal be consulted on properly, but also that there should be consultation as a routine on all possible change, that this should include listening to members (not just giving presentations) and that there should be as a matter of routine transparent and freely accessible paper trailing of views from every part of the UK and every part of the RCN membership.

Communication between members was greatly inhibited by the denial of access to members' email addresses. Forum chairs were not alone in complaining: there were complaints from secretaries of branches who had no access to their members' email addresses, for example, even for the essential task of giving details of the next branch meeting; they were repeatedly told that access was precluded by the Data Protection

Act (which is untrue). The issue was raised at Congress 2013, and I was concerned that no mention was included in the Report of Council at Congress 2014 on action taken since then. Since I did not intend to be present in person at Congress 2014, I sent an email to the Chair of Council asking what action had been taken in respect of the issue. I was surprised but delighted when my email was read out to Congress, and the Chair said, to considerable applause, that he gave a personal commitment to sorting this out. In July the Council set up a project team that would report back to Council – in a year's time. From correspondence with the Information Commissioner's Office I was able to show that there was no barrier in the Data Protection Act to sharing such information within the organisation; that since members had already given their consent to 'the RCN' in an opt-out system, no extra consent was necessary; and that any such ban was an internal decision within the organisation. It was clear that members had been blatantly misled.

Everyone recognised the need to save money – the problem was the way in which it was done. This ruthless imposition of central control included suppression of any criticism of the organisation, and strict control of information. The relevant committees discussed their business in a private session and requests for copies of minutes were repeatedly rejected. The Council policies on openness and transparency were removed from the website, and in spite of commitments made at the time, have never been replaced. Postings on the Discussion Zone that attempted to criticise decisions or raise questions about what was happening were rapidly and repeatedly removed as 'outside the Acceptable Use Policy'.

In a personal note to me, one fellow activist neatly summed up the process: 'Subsequent postings remind me of another trend I have noticed. The leadership makes certain proposals, there is an outcry, and some members take to the streets of the Discussion Zone with their metaphorical placards and hold a virtual protest. The leadership responds with carefully crafted responses. The protesting members are reassured, and the train carrying the implementation rattles on to its destination. In due course there is further weeping and wailing and gnashing of teeth, when it seems that that which was implemented does not seem to correspond with the interpretation that some of the former protesters placed on the clarification that the leadership provided to address the clear misunderstanding of the proposals as originally communicated. In due course, everything settles down and members do what nurses always do, they try to make the new system work. Eventually it seems to move in the direction of what they wanted all along.'

A drop in engagement

One result of these changes has been a dramatic drop in member engagement. The issue was raised as a Matter for Discussion at Congress 2013. The indicator discussed was participation in elections and voting turnouts. Voting turnouts are never high either in the RCN or elsewhere, but there are some clues in the different rates for different kinds of elections and votes. Probably the most relevant indicator is voting at AGMs, in particular on matters related to subscriptions. In the 2000 AGM 45 000 members voted on the various resolutions. By 2013, the number of votes had fallen to 261 – less than one in 1500 members. By 2014, in the elections for members of the regional boards, in seven of the nine English regions and one of the three Celtic countries there were not enough candidates to hold an election, and a new call for nominations had to be made. The AGM of my local branch was abandoned as inquorate as just four people, including myself, turned up. For the 2015 Council elections the turnout was just 5%.

Many commentators have noted that the decline had accelerated over the past decade. Several blame 'apathy', but do not explain it. I am sure that apathy plays a part, but I believe that this is exacerbated by increasingly poor communication and exclusion from decision making, leading to a vicious circle of 'learned helplessness' in which, in accordance with the new governance structure, the less that members are allowed to do the less they do, and then the less they want to do, thus producing a downward spiral of less and less engagement and participation.

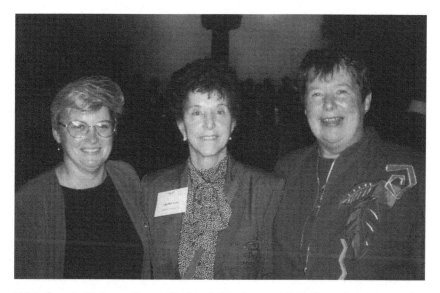

With Connie Delaney (l) and Virginia Saba, doyens of nursing informatics in the USA

CHAPTER 12: THE INFORMATION IN NURSING FORUM

After my term of office as President was over, it was the development of health informatics in the UK, and in particular in Wales, that brought me back to the RCN as an activist. Back in 1993, during a Telenurse workshop held in Greece, I met Anne Casey, a paediatric nurse who had become interested in the development of standardised terminology. Anne was working as the leader of the Nursing Terms Project to identify the terms to be included in the Read codes, which were being developed as the standardised terminology to be used by GPs. On a glorious bus ride from Athens to Delphi, when we should have been admiring the scenery, we spent the whole time discussing the nature of nursing and how it could be best represented in computerised information systems. We discovered that we shared the same concept of nursing as 'knowledge work', to which information management is central, rather than the prevailing concept of 'nursing as doing'. We discussed how we could get the RCN involved, and agreed that we needed a membership group and a member of staff to focus the work.

Using the RCN forums

We decided that a good way to get members involved in informatics was to engage them through a Forum. During the mid-1990s the old Computers in Nursing Forum, which had fallen into disuse because it was perceived as being for 'techies' only, was revitalised as the Information in Nursing Group, shortened deliberately to 'the IN Group'. The title Information in Nursing Group was intended to make explicit the message that information management is the business of every nurse and integral to every nurse's practice. In the introduction to our first publication, which we entitled *Putting Information at the Heart of Nursing Care: How IT is Set to Revolutionise Health Care and the NHS*, we wrote:

Welcome to the 21st century!
Information technology (IT) has become part of our everyday lives. [...] Just as surely as it's made a world of difference to commerce and industry, IT will change the practice of every nurse, health visitor, midwife and health care assistant. IT will also affect nursing students while on clinical placements. Nurses will have to learn new skills to use this technology and if IT is to fulfil its promise, then nurses need to be involved in telling the systems developers and vendors what information these systems must contain. If nurses don't do this, other people will, and nurses may find themselves using systems that increase their workload without benefiting patients.

By 2002, the information management and technology (IM&T) agenda in all four countries in the UK was developing rapidly. In Wales a series of taskforces was developed to take forward the new post-devolution strategy for the NHS, and I secured membership of the group concerned with the development of information systems which resulted, in 2003, in the first Welsh strategy for the development of IM&T, 'Informing Healthcare'.

Joining the IN Forum steering committee

I realised that to keep in touch with what was happening outside Wales, I needed to become more actively involved in the IN Forum and in 2004 I stood for election to the steering committee. I was elected initially as representative for Wales, and then, in August 2005, became Chair. I was supported by a very enthusiastic steering committee: Bernice Baker (who became Vice-Chairperson), Paul Linsley, Elizabeth Hunter, Katie Farnell, and later Alison Wallis (representing Scotland, who later became Chair and later still joined the RCN staff as Nurse Adviser), Mike Dunne (representing Northern Ireland), and by our part-time Nurse Adviser Sharon Levy. These people became close friends as well as colleagues who stood by me through thick and thin – in particular the 'thin', which was to come.

The work programme was huge because the NHS IM&T programmes in all four countries of the UK were accelerating rapidly. As soon as I became Chair I realised that if we were to achieve anything we needed to sort out some ways of working. I was disturbed to find that the Headquarters' support for Forums was inadequate. For example, although I was responsible for the Forum's budget, which came in the form of an annual grant plus any money we could raise from activities such as conferences, the financial information from Headquarters that was necessary to manage it was hopelessly poor. I therefore ended up working with the Forum Chairs Group to correct this. We wanted to involve as many Forum members as possible in the work, but our only means of communication with members was our biannual newsletter. The Headquarters' IT systems were primitive, so Sharon began to develop a members' Listserv so those members who wanted to be involved could keep in touch by email. In addition to this, Bernice, using her position at the Centre for Practice Development at Bournemouth University, established a JISCMail facility.

One challenge was to ensure that there was a nursing voice in as many of the various groups and organisations that were springing up as possible. Each member of the steering committee, and some of the activists who had joined the Listserv, took responsibility for liaising with one or more of these groups and submitting a report to each steering committee meeting. The time commitment was considerable, and all the other committee members had full time 'day jobs'. Since I was now retired I was luckily able to give the time the committee needed.

Challenges: Lack of interest and readiness

The biggest challenge was to get nurses – not least the RCN 'establishment' – to recognise that information management (we always stressed that this was the key concept and that IT was merely the vehicle for achieving it) was central to nursing practice and needed to be integrated into every aspect of the RCN's work. In 1996, following my sabbatical to the USA, when I had written a paper entitled 'Information is power: How the American Nurses Association manages information', no interest had been shown in information management. A decade later within the RCN only Sharon and Anne had experience and understanding of ehealth, especially standardised

185

terminology and electronic patient records, which were the particular focus of our attention. We argued that ehealth was in the same position now as research had been a decade earlier – still viewed as a specialist activity relevant to few – and that it needed the same kind of organisational and financial investment by the RCN as research had received in order to achieve the same kind of culture change. We argued the case in meetings with the Research Society (who had not yet recognised the research resources contained in information systems) and the Management Forum, and met with very limited success. We tried to get items onto the Congress agenda and repeatedly failed. We continued to speak at the conferences and meetings of other forums, and Sharon and Anne continued to lobby internally though staff meetings.

My immediate concern was the lack of readiness of nurses in Wales with regards to information management. My involvement with Informing Healthcare and as a non-executive director of the Carmarthenshire NHS Trust had demonstrated the lack of awareness among nurses and the belief among other disciplines (the specialist informaticists and the medical profession) that nurses did not need to be involved. At a nursing conference in Wales back in 1995 I had said 'In future nursing will be defined, managed and controlled by the information about it held in computerised information systems', and been laughed off the platform. A paper I had prepared for the Welsh Nursing and Midwifery Advisory Committee had suffered the same fate. My retirement conference in September 2003 had attracted participants from all over the world – except from Wales.

The all-Wales group: Enwi

My first thought was to develop a regional subgroup of the IN Forum in Wales, but I soon realised that there was not enough interest to do so. So in November 2004 we organised a 1-day conference in Cardiff with the title 'Informing Healthcare, Informing Nursing'; the final session of the day was given over to the launch of a new all-Wales group, which was not limited to RCN members, and could provide support and educational resources to all nurses in Wales. It was conceived as a 'virtual' organisation, using the ehealth nurses network that had already been established by Bernice for nurses in England. A coordinating committee was formed consisting of a representative of each of the nursing organisations operating in Wales (RCN, Royal College of Midwives, Community Practitioners and Health Visitors Association, and British Computer Society) plus a representative from the Chief Nursing Officer's office and one from Informing Healthcare.

Following a competition among those who wanted to join, the term 'enwi', the Welsh word for 'to name', was chosen as the organisation's name.

I agreed to act as Chair of Enwi for the first few months while we got established, and then handed over to Rodney Hughes. Rodney was one of my former PhD students who had since become a lecturer at Bangor University. He, along with his colleague Dave Lloyd, had started a small group for interested nurses in North Wales. When Gwyn Thomas was appointed Director of Informing Healthcare in 2005, we were waiting on his doorstep to let him know what we were doing and to lobby for the appointment of a nurse to his team.

In October 2005 we organised a conference in North Wales on the theme 'Naming Nursing in an Information Age', and in November 2006 we held the third workshop in Cardiff in conjunction with Bournemouth University's Centre for Practice Development on 'From Paper to Electronic Records – What is Needed for Nursing?' In her role as lecturer–practitioner, Bernice already had considerable experience of running workshops and conferences. Without the financial and administrative support of the Centre for Practice Development, however, we could not have achieved what we did. The centrepiece of the third workshop was Rodney and Dave's presentation of 'A conceptual model for nursing information', which was subsequently published in the *International Journal of Terminology and Classification*, and presented at international conferences in USA (NANDA) and Amsterdam (Association for Common European Nursing Diagnoses and Outcomes, ACENDIO).

At the 2006 NANDA conference held in Chicago, Rodney and I presented an account of the development of Enwi under the title 'Enwi: the story of a "Nurses for Nurses" collaboration in Wales'. We donated a Welsh love spoon to the fundraising auction at the conference dinner... and raised more money by our rendition of the Welsh national anthem (in Welsh) than was raised by the spoon! Sadly, soon afterwards Rodney became ill, and he died in February 2007. Enwi kept going with Dave as its Chair for a few more years, but following Rodney's death and the retirement of Dave and Bernice it gradually faded away.

European level: ACENDIO

Progress was much faster at international level than it was within the UK. Following the First European Conference on Nursing Diagnoses held in Copenhagen in 1993, ACENDIO was established in 1995. I became the first Honorary Secretary and then President. Secretariat services were provided by the RCN through Anne Casey, and the RCN funded our attendance at board

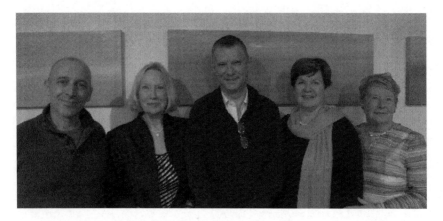

Presidents of ACENDIO: Fintan Sheerin (Ireland), Randi Mortensen (Denmark), Walter Sermeus (Belgium), Kaija Saranto (Finland), and June.

meetings. The ACENDIO Board met two or three times a year in the various member countries. We produced a regular newsletter and organised biennial conferences in Brussels, Amsterdam, Helsinki, Bled, Berlin, Madeira and Dublin. We collaborated with NANDA and AENDE (the Spanish-speaking association) and attended their conferences. The biennial conferences were (and still are) highly successful and well attended by participants from all over Europe. In 2015 ACENDIO held a special conference in Switzerland to celebrate its tenth conference.

An expert in ehealth?

Meanwhile, as a result of all this activity, I was becoming recognised at national and international level as an expert in ehealth. This recognition went far beyond my actual level of expertise. In 2005 I was appointed (the only nurse) to a Royal Society working group to consider the impact of ICT on healthcare now and for the future. For a year I had the privilege of working alongside the country's best brains in informatics. Our report was published in 2006 with the title *Digital Healthcare: the Impact of Information and Communication Technologies on Health and Healthcare*. I was invited to give the opening plenary lecture at the huge international informatics conference Nursing Informatics 2006, held that year in Seoul, Korea. In 2008 the theme of the Commonwealth Health Ministers Meeting was ehealth, and the RCN was commissioned to prepare a background paper on the human resources implications of ehealth. I wrote the paper and prepared the PowerPoint presentation.

Breakthrough at the RCN

In the RCN the breakthrough came in May 2007 when, following considerable lobbying, we achieved a meeting with the (then new) General Secretary. In my briefing paper for the meeting I wrote:

The position of the UK in the international informatics arena is frankly embarrassing – a few individuals held in very high regard internationally with no recognition or support in the UK, which is miles behind other countries. Preparation for ehealth, especially for [electronic patient records], will take time – but it is urgent because IT is happening now and will not wait. There are major educational needs (not just computer skills training) and the RCN has a responsibility to assist its members. There are key policy issues [...]. The RCN currently has no policy or statement of strategic intent on ehealth and (amazingly) does not refer to it in such strategic planning documents as it does have. [...] There is no clear lead for ehealth within the RCN – doubtless a reflection of its low priority.

I summarised the key messages as:

The integration of ehealth into nursing practice is a professional not an IT issue [...]. ehealth will impinge on every aspect of nursing practice. If the RCN does not handle it proactively now, it will have to cope reactively later in the form of members' trade union needs, e.g. job losses. [...] If we used it properly it would provide solutions to many current priorities, e.g. could demonstrate as opposed to merely asserting the value of specialist nurses; save nurses time; greatly improve the efficiency of the RCN, etc. So instead of being low priority on the RCN's agenda, it needs to be top priority as a pre-requisite for achieving other priorities (e.g. future nurse workforce work, RCN financial management, etc).

I quoted a remark made by Connie Holloran, then CEO of the ICN: 'If the profession in the shape of its professional association fails to take a lead on a professional issue, someone else, usually government, will fill the vacuum.'

We proposed that in order to kick-start the process, a workshop should be held involving both RCN staff and IN Forum members. A 2-day workshop was held in Cardiff in January 2008, and as is my wont, the workshop had an internal and an external agenda. The internal agenda was to get together staff from different departments of the RCN to improve

189

their awareness and understanding of the relevance of ehealth to the work of the RCN, and to establish a way of working in which Forum members and staff could work together. The external agenda or task was to prepare the policy statements and guidance for members that were urgently needed. Pre-workshop documentation was prepared and circulated. Following some plenary introduction, participants worked in two groups. One group worked on developing web-based guidance for members; the second group worked on publications for guidance to members and draft policies. Finally, in the plenary session, the workshop reviewed the general direction and overall plan for the development of ehealth within the RCN's strategic and operational plans. We defined the IN Forum's action plan for 2008–9, and agreed to set up an eHealth Programme Board that would draw together the work of all departments and make it all happen.

We achieved another breakthrough at Congress 2008: ehealth and the work of the IN Forum were explicitly referred to in both the Council report and the General Secretary's speech. Our fringe meeting, under the title 'Computer says no. Are you bovvered?', was very well attended. Whether this was because of the strange title, or the prize of a MP3 player for one lucky attendee donated by our sponsor Map of Medicine, I do not know. At long last we managed to get an item onto the agenda. Item number 22 read: 'that this meeting of Congress supports the implementation and use of telehealth services in the community for patients with long term conditions.' It did not matter the motion referred to 'telehealth' (remote delivery of health care) and the title it was given in the agenda papers was 'telecare' (that is, assistive technology in people's homes), although this was an indicator of the level of ignorance within the RCN about ehealth. What mattered was that it gave an opportunity to speak about ehealth in general. As it was, few speakers stuck either to the motion or its title.

In my 'Letter from the Chair' in the Spring 2008 issue of the IN Forum Newsletter, I wrote:

Exciting times! At last the message that we have been promoting for years is getting through: ehealth is an integral part of nursing and must therefore be an integral part of the work of the RCN! When General Secretary and Chief Executive Dr Peter Carter joined the meeting of the Information in Nursing Forum Steering Committee in October he confirmed his support for the work we are doing and agreed that ehealth should be moved further up the RCN's agenda. As a result, ehealth is now listed as one of the seven priorities for the RCN during the next year and should therefore be included in the operational plans of every RCN department. We have an emerging RCN ehealth Programme whose Programme Board will develop and co-ordinate the RCN's activities in this field. The Board will include both staff and forum members, and a member of RCN Council. Jackie Cheeseborough, Head of Information and Knowledge Development in the RCN Institute, has been named as the RCN strategic lead on ehealth to work alongside Sharon Levy and Anne Casey, our nurse advisers. Angela Perrett (currently head of library services in Wales) has been appointed as a part time project manager to make sure that it all happens.

Meanwhile we were supporting several specific projects. The first, an investigation of the emergent professional issues experienced by nurses when working in an ehealth environment, led by Bernice, sought to explore the professional and ethical issues of importance to nursing that were emerging as a result of the introduction of information and communications technology into the NHS in order to identify areas where RCN policy and guidance to members needed to be developed. Using focus groups and key informant interviews, its main finding was that there was an enormous gap between the vision of the potential of ehealth as it was enthusiastically articulated by the ehealth leaders, and the reality experienced by front-line nurses. The second project, led by David Baker, the student member of our steering group, consisted of two phases: an online survey of student nurses that sought a UK-wide snapshot of their current experiences of ehealth, followed by a workshop for key people representing areas such as higher education, clinical practice placements, education commissioners, NHS IT programmes, chief nursing officers, and the Nursing & Midwifery Council, to discuss the survey findings and make recommendations about the key actions to be undertaken to resolve the challenges exposed. Our most ambitious and important project was to develop a 'model system' or 'template' for the nursing content of an electronic patient record that could be offered to suppliers to ensure that the systems they developed really supported nursing practice as opposed to merely administrative requirements. Our work-plan for 2009–10 read as follows:

4-year vision: All RCN members are engaged appropriately in ehealth, supported by an organisation that is recognised nationally and internationally as a leader in the field.

Programme objectives:

There were 40 items in our 2008–9 operational plan, and the new rules for forums required that for every item we had to prepare a fully documented and costed business plan. I worked day and night on the documentation required. The agenda was huge, but the workshop gave us confidence that we could achieve it. We were on the crest of a wave.

We had established an eHealth Programme Board that included IN Forum representatives working alongside staff. We had a very heavy programme of representing the RCN at meetings of other organisations working on ehealth, several specific projects in progress, including one concerned with developing a template to include nursing in the rapidly-developing electronic patient records that were beginning to come into use in the NHS; and we were planning a major conference for which we had secured a world-famous international speaker.

Everything was finally coming together. And then came the crash. There was no warning, no consultation, and no flexibility. Our IN Forum budget was removed. Our carefully prepared operational plan for the next year was axed. Our pre-arranged Steering Group meetings were cancelled. The work of the IN Forum was abruptly halted.

CHAPTER 13: THE END OF THE LOVE AFFAIR

It is hard to write about something as painful as the end of a love affair. I was devastated by what was happening to the Forums and in particular to the IN Forum, which I had worked so hard to develop. At the time, writing down everything that happened was cathartic and comforting. Reflecting on it much later, however, opens old wounds and re-ignites the pain. The events described in this chapter are documented in greater detail in the archives of the Discussion Zone, the Forum Chairs' listserv, in emails and other correspondence. Sadly, copyright law and the threat of litigation mean that many of the most significant parts have had to be omitted here; they are, however, available in the RCN Archives so that future historians can better understand what happened to me and to others during this dark period.

At first I tried to make the new rules work. I knew that change was needed, and I had been deeply involved in the work of the Forum Chairs to put things right. With my steering committee I tried to rearrange and amalgamate meetings to re-plan our activities. My efforts were interpreted as 'manipulating the system'. All our work of the previous 3 years was just wiped out.

The trigger for my personal crisis – stupid as triggers often are – was the new expenses policy that forbade overnight accommodation, accompanied by a directive that meetings must start at 11am and finish at 4pm (with no consideration of where people were coming from or what was the purpose or agenda for the meeting). The two policies were closely inter-related, but for me the row was not about money: the issue was about power and control.

The new expenses policy was sensible, but its implementation was chaotic. The policy itself wisely used words such as 'normally' or 'wherever possible', but the staff whom the members were instructed to contact reported that they were instructed to refuse overnight accommodation at all costs, even where same-day travel required a member to leave home at 4 am, or in my own case 6 am. This was a classic example of the command and control management style and the rigid approach to rules that dominated the whole change programme. The system took no account of members' circumstances such as the off-duty requirements of their day jobs or their inability to specify off duty arrangements far in advance. Members complained that staff made unrealistic bookings based on inadequate knowledge, and that the agency that was contracted to supply tickets made costly mistakes and did not always obtain the cheapest tickets.

All Forums were affected by the rationalisation and Forum chairs protested individually and collectively, but the rigidity of the interpretation of the policy hit the IN Forum particularly hard because of our huge work programme and because, responding to Council policy to ensure UK-wide representation, our steering committee included members from Scotland and Northern Ireland, who were refused overnight accommodation and expected to use same-day arrangements. Our Scottish member wrote to Peter Carter describing how the new policy affected her: it meant that for the forthcoming meeting she would have to leave home at 4 am, would not arrive home until 10.30 pm, and would have to be in work as usual early the next morning. She pointed out that while she appreciated that the RCN had to be accountable to its members for the cost of meetings, there was also an obligation to those members who were helping the RCN to provide a service by making sure that they can do so effectively and without any negative effect on their ability to function. She requested that the RCN reconsider this policy and gave assurance that any changes were monitored and audited and the results made available to the Forums.

To no avail. Other Forum chairs also protested: the email traffic on the Forum chairs' Listserv was vitriolic.

I did not ask for or expect any favours, but I expected the policy to be interpreted sensibly. For me the rule meant getting up getting up at 5 am and leaving home before 6 am for a train journey that would get me to London barely in time to start chairing a meeting whose agenda I knew we could not possibly finish by 4 pm, followed by a return journey that might involve a long wait at Paddington Station for the train specified by the booking. At the age of 68 it was just too much. I was able to demonstrate that the travel arrangements that I could make including an overnight stay were considerably cheaper than those being arranged by the RCN's travel agency for same-day travel. The Director of the Governance Support Unit, which was responsible for the policy and its implementation, was eventually forced to concede that I was right, but justified the previous refusals by saying that she wanted to check for herself.

I tried desperately to find a way of managing our enormous work programme within the new constraints. Our Nurse Adviser Sharon Levy decided that his position was untenable; he resigned and was not replaced. In his absence the work of the Forum fell on me: soon I was working 2 or 3 days a week on Forum business. I was glad to do the work. I had an enthusiastic and supportive team for a steering committee, which now included members from all four countries that make up the UK. This met a Council policy that few other forums had managed to implement.

The new rules required submission of a 'contingency bid' for funding for travel or any other activity. Each bid required a fully costed business case, which I spent many hours preparing. In their report to Council, the Forums Governance Group noted that 95% of bids had been accepted; however, all seven of ours were rejected. The reasons given for rejection were specious, for example that the Forums Governance Group could not fund forum chairs to come to London for meetings with their co-ordinator because these should happen when forum chairs were at Cavendish Square for other meetings. However, the rules meant that there were no meetings other than Steering Committees, and since even these were time-limited, there was now no opportunity to add a second meeting on the same day.

The decision that most angered me, however, was the award of £20 000 to another Forum for an ehealth project that had not been discussed by either the IN Forum or the eHealth Programme Board and conflicted with the agreed RCN policy against individual stand-alone systems. Rightly or wrongly, I felt that I and the IN Forum were becoming the target of a personal vendetta.

The battle continued throughout the summer. I became more and more distressed. By September I decided that I had had enough.

On 4 September I wrote to Peter Carter, setting out in detail the events of the previous few months. The letter was not even acknowledged.

I decided to go to the AGM to be held in Liverpool on 20 October and say publicly just how I felt about what was happening to the Forums. I had prepared an impassioned speech, which I showed to some colleagues. Peter Carter heard about it and begged me not to deliver it. I yielded to his advice, and agreed instead to write to him about my complaints. My letter of 23 October said that I just could not take any more. I said that as Forum Chair I expected to take responsibility for managing my Forum's business within agreed policies and procedures, and did not expect my decisions, which were based on careful and rational planning, to be overturned without even any consultation with me. I said that I could not work that way. I pointed out that Forum Chairs were not naughty children, and to be treated like naughty children was patronising and insulting.

A week later Peter Carter responded telling me that the Chair of Council and Chair of the Forums Governance Committee had agreed that for as long as I remained a Forum Chair my overnight expenses would be met when required, 'on health and age grounds'. However, this was conditional on my compliance with all other aspects of the policy including the use of advance tickets on specific trains, and that I did not use my presence in London the night before as a reason for starting my Forum meetings earlier or for asking for overnight accommodation for other members of the committee.

I felt demeaned and insulted and was deeply offended by the imputation that I had abused my own position to ask for overnight accommodation for others (the two members of the Steering Committee who came from Scotland and Northern Ireland). In any case I had already resigned as Forum Chair, so the 'concession' was meaningless.

However, there was no letup in the pressure.

When putting together my last 'Chairman's Letter' for the IN Forum Newsletter, I wrote: 'The past few months have been a difficult time for forums. They are currently undergoing radical change to their composition and in their ways of working. The number of forums is being reduced, mainly by a process of mergers and rationalisation.... However, in future, all members will be limited to joining only one forum instead of, as at present, as many as they wish. Meanwhile the RCN Forums Governance Group has introduced new rules about how forums are managed – steering committee meetings are now reduced to two per year, are limited in time, and all expenditure has to be authorised by the Forums Governance Group. It is because I cannot work as Forum Chair within what I perceive as a straitjacket that I have decided to resign my post.'

I submitted this text to the Editor (a member of the IN Forum Steering Committee), who approved it, prepared it for printing, and sent it back to me for final proofing. I returned it to her, assuming that this was how it would appear in the final published version. When we received our copies of the Newsletter some weeks later, however, both the Editor and I were shocked to see that, without any reference to either of us, the text had been changed. My first paragraph, my explanation of why I was resigning as Chair, and my description of the changes, had been deleted. The revised piece was moved from the front page to an inside page and the space now released by this change was given over to an advertisement for a different forum's forthcoming conference.

The final straw, however, was the email sent to me by the Chair of the Forums Governance Group, on 17 November, which 'explained' why the Forums Governance Group could not approve either the original or the revised proposal for our proposed away-day at the beginning of December. It gave as its reason the 'lack of respect' that we had shown for the decision making process. It said that she had 'seen an email', in which she had interpreted the use of the words 'a creative solution' to mean a manipulative attempt 'get round the rules'.

The email in question, which had been intended only for our steering committee, sought to find a 'creative' way of doing things differently in order to get better value for money. The plan was to combine a meeting of the steering committee with a project meeting about the SNOMED project. The money to support the away-day was already in the Forum's previously-approved budget, but the only meetings now permitted were meetings to support specific projects. The purpose of the away-day was to plan a strategy for achieving the Forum's commitments within the new arrangements that were being imposed, and the continuing failure (after three attempts) to appoint to the Nurse Adviser post, which had now been vacant for almost a year. We were trying to find a way out of the impossible position the IN Forum was in and identify a future for it. My attempt to reduce costs by the 'creative solution' of combining a steering committee with a SNOMED meeting was rejected as 'a manipulative move by this forum to get their own way'.

The IN Forum Steering Committee met on 6–7 December at our own expense, because the Forums Governance Group had refused to authorise the travel costs. We considered alternative plans to maintain such activities as we could. We also considered withdrawing from the RCN altogether.

A meeting with Peter Carter was arranged. I assumed that its purpose was to find a way forward for the IN Forum. I was wrong. On 12 December I received a letter from Peter Carter stating that the purpose for wishing to meet with me was to bring to my attention that a number of members and staff had expressed concern over the email traffic and correspondence on the Discussion Zone over the recent period. As a consequence the matter had been discussed at the recent meeting of the Council Executive Team, the outcome of which was that this required a formal investigation. I recognised the final sentence, that I was entitled to be accompanied by a friend or representative of my choice at the meeting, as the wording used in disciplinary proceedings.

Acrimonious exchanges

The meeting was scheduled for 5 February 2009. Sylvia Denton, former RCN President, agreed to accompany me. I went away for a holiday over Christmas, and expected more information to be available on my return on 13 January. There was nothing. I wrote again on 14 January, requesting information about the allegations that were being made against me. On 23 January I received a letter that set out the following 'charges':

- My attendance at the October 2007 and February 2008 Council meetings when the PMS proposals were discussed;
- My part in the interviews for the ehealth adviser post at the end of 2008;
- A number of my postings on the Discussion Zone;
- My complaint against the decisions of the Forums Governance Group in respect of my contingency bids and the way I responded to these not being approved;
- My draft editorial for the IN Group newsletter;
- My working relationships with a range of members and staff.'

To these were added on the day:
- 'An article I wrote in *The Guardian* in May 2004.'

I was stunned. I checked with the then Chair of Council whether she remembered anything untoward about the two Council meetings referred to, which had taken place more than a year previously; she could identify nothing. I agreed that I had been premature in telling my steering committee the previous October that we had, for the third time, failed to appoint a nurse adviser – although there was no breach of confidentiality and it had not been mentioned at the time. I looked at recent postings on the Discussion Zone, at my emails to the Forums Governance Group about the rejection of our contingency bids, and my editorial announcing my resignation as Forum Chair and could find nothing 'offensive'. And I could not see the relevance of an article I had written for *The Guardian* newspaper in 2004 – 5 years previously.

Nevertheless I hoped that the proposed meeting would be an opportunity to clear the air, to agree that both sides had made mistakes for which we would apologise, and to enable us to 'move on'. I was wrong. The agenda had changed from dealing with my complaints to making allegations about me. There was no opportunity to discuss any of my concerns. Instead it was a concerted attack on me. It changed my role from plaintiff to defendant. I was distraught. That meeting marked the nadir in the already deteriorating relationship and a significant turning point.

The acrimonious correspondence continued. In each letter I re-iterated that all I wanted was that the allegations made against me, which had not been substantiated, should be withdrawn. It never happened. On 22 July 2009 I wrote: 'In view of the refusal to withdraw the allegations that have been made about me which I believe to be untrue and which damage my professional reputation and my standing within the RCN, I am now formally requesting a full investigation of my complaints.' My complaints were:

■ 'The manner of the application to me and members of my Steering Committee of the RCN expenses policy;
■ The decisions of the FGG relating to the Information in Nursing Forum;
■ The behaviour of the Chair of the FGG towards me culminating in her email to me dated 17th November 2008;
■ The failure to consider these complaints, and the substitution for them of further allegations about me.'

On 26 August (i.e. a month later), Peter Carter wrote to say that my complaints had been investigated 'in accordance with our agreed procedures'. I was not involved in the process or even informed that this was happening. The complaint about the way the expenses issue was handled was 'investigated' by the Council Review Group, who had confirmed the decisions of which I complained; the complaints about the FGG were 'investigated' by the FGG; the final complaint was not mentioned at all. Some complaints procedure!

This letter was, however, significant in other respects and in reply I wrote:

When I read your letter of 26th August at last the penny dropped – it was a eureka moment!... For the first time in all our correspondence, your letter of 26th August makes explicit your views about the RCN as a membership organisation and the roles of members within it. ... it is now clear that we were never going to agree, and that in future the RCN will be a very different kind of organisation from the one that I have been proud to serve for more than forty years.

Five years on: the wounds re-open

Over the following years the wounds did gradually heal, albeit with considerable scar tissue, and I thought I had put things behind me. Until in April 2013, almost 5 years later, I received an email from a Frank McKenna, whom I did not know but subsequently discovered was a management consultant acting for the RCN, stating that he had been asked to make contact with me to set up a time to meet with me in advance of a meeting between Dr Peter Carter and myself. In the hope that a facilitated meeting might finally achieve closure I cautiously agreed. In order to prepare for our meeting I asked him to send me the following information:

1. Why now – 5 years after the relevant events?
2. What is the brief that you have been given?
3. What outcome do you/Peter Carter expect to achieve?
4. What is the agenda for our meeting?

In the emails that followed over the next 7 months I repeated the same questions. No answer was forthcoming, until on 28 November 2013, a week before the scheduled meeting, Peter Carter wrote to me saying that he wanted to re-emphasise that the current process was set up by him personally to address comments made by me about him on the Discussion Zone on 10 June 2012... He stressed that the meeting was about the comments about members that I had attributed to him in June 2012.

On searching through old files on my computer, I found the offending posting and the correspondence that had followed it. The thread, started by another RCN member, was entitled 'Governance Review' and focused on the protests made at Congress about the imposition, without consultation of changes, to the constitutions of RCN Boards. The same day another member had posted a message suggesting that conspiracy theorists might see this as another way to take power from the elected membership and place that power in the hands of a selected few. I had joined the discussion, repeating my definition of a member-led organisation as one in which members were fully engaged in running their organisation through the processes of representative democracy, and drawing attention to a letter in which Peter Carter had said that the only function of members in a membership organisation (apart from providing the money to fund staff and their activities) was to elect the Council. Peter Carter misread my posting, as claiming that he had said that the only function of members was to fund staff – he said that he considered this to be demeaning and simply not accurate. He considered that since I had produced no evidence to support my claim it was perfectly reasonable of him to ask me to withdraw the remarks.

After several postponements the facilitated meeting was eventually held on 6 December 2013 – 8 months after the original request. It was agreed that there should be an exchange of letters in which I would apologise for offence caused and would in future refrain from such remarks, and Peter Carter would state that the allegations made against me were found to be unsubstantiated and were withdrawn. Three rounds of drafts of these letters were written and circulated; each time the sentence that stated the 'allegations made against me were found to be unsubstantiated and were withdrawn' was removed. In spite of repeated requests, no explanation for this removal was given. I refused to sign any letter that did not contain this sentence.

By April 2014, after a whole year of prevarication, my patience had run out. I felt I had been thoroughly messed about, and I issued an ultimatum: 'Either you will agree to this inclusion or you won't: if I do not hear from you within fourteen days I will assume that this correspondence is closed.' There was no reply from Peter Carter, but some weeks later Frank McKenna replied, asking for one more attempt. I agreed. In September I received an email from him saying that Peter Carter had now agreed, but in return both Peter and I would be asked to sign a non-disclosure agreement. I refused.

There has been no reply, and I assume that the correspondence is closed.

An ending

Although to the casual observer this might seem something of a storm in a teacup, it affected me deeply. For months the events of 2008–9 dominated every minute of my thinking. I found it hard to sleep, and when I did sleep there were nightmares and flashbacks to the meeting of February 2009. The only thing that sustained me was the wise words of Tina Donnelly, Director of RCN Wales, spoken during a tearful encounter after receiving the latest email: 'Remember, no-one can take away what you have already achieved.'

It is a sad story, but the saddest part is that as I contacted colleagues and friends who were around at the time, just to check for any inaccuracies in this account, I found that several of them – former presidents, members of Council, and Forum chairs – had had similar experiences and felt a similar disenchantment with the organisation that they too had served faithfully. It was a dark period in the history of the College.

Green shoots

As Dylan Thomas once wrote: 'Though lovers be lost, love shall not.'

The RCN is still in my blood. Trust can, and I believe, will be rebuilt, but it will take time. I remain a member, participating as actively as I can in Wales, where I have always received friendship and support. I attend branch meetings and participate in branch social activities. I have recently been elected to lead the group that represents the RCN in the National Pensioners Convention. I remain nominally a member of the IN Forum (now renamed the eHealth Forum), although for several years there have been no communications to members and no opportunities for active participation. In practice the IN forum no longer exists. I have established a Trust to provide travel scholarships for Welsh nurses in an attempt to share the benefits I was given throughout my nursing career through learning about nursing in other countries.

And I have taken new lovers.... Sigma Theta Tau International Honor Society of Nursing (STTI) is an international nursing organisation whose mission is 'advancing world health and celebrating nursing excellence in scholarship, leadership, and service'. I helped to establish a chapter in Wales, served for 2 years on the International Board of Directors, and in 2012 organised its first European conference.

I have re-joined the St John Ambulance Brigade, in which 60 years ago I was a cadet and which was probably the trigger for my interest in nursing. I now serve as a member of the West Glamorgan Council and as County Nursing Adviser, as well as being a member of my local (Mumbles) Division. I continue my commitment to the cause of older people as a trustee of Age Cymru, and in helping to establish a local 'befriending' service.

I maintain my academic links through membership of the Council of Swansea University, where I am a Professor Emeritus. Swansea University now counts among the top 30 research universities in the UK and has received numerous accolades, including winner of the Student Nursing Times Award

2014 as Pre-registration Nurse Education Provider of the Year. I am proud to be associated with it.

In addition to my nursing links, I am blessed by a loving family: a wonderful husband, two children and five lovely grandchildren. I am enjoying life and all its blessings.

In *The Guardian* article that I wrote in May 2004, which was the subject of one of the complaints made against me, I asked: 'Can an organisation as large and complex as the RCN be turned around?' In answer, I wrote: 'I have seen it do so before and I believe that it can now.'

In 2015 there are, I believe, some hopeful signs. In 2014 we got a new Chair of Council and in 2015 a new Chief Executive – an opportunity to develop a new leadership style and organisational culture. The 'top of the office' management team has been restructured. The Governance Support Unit is no longer an independent Directorate but is managed by the Director of Finance and Business Enablement. There is a new post of Director of Nursing Policy and Practice who will be a member of the top management team. The Annual Report for 2014–5 shows a dramatic change from previous years: 'Being a professional organisation' is listed as the first of the Council's priorities – ahead of 'Being a trade union' and 'Being a value for money organisation'. There is a commitment to knowledge development, albeit through knowledge transfer rather than knowledge creation through original research. A new website will provide for interaction between ordinary members and their elected representatives.

Having sorted out the problem of access to members' email addresses, the Chair of Council has stated that his next personal priority is to improve member engagement. In 2015 for the first time in 6 years some Forum chairs are being elected instead of being appointed. In the light of the low turnout in the 2015 Council elections (average 5%) there is clearly work to be done. Work has begun on redeveloping the Forums and I am assured that all Forum members, not just the appointed steering committees and their chairs, will be consulted.

And in the end, if the RCN is to become once again the world's premier professional association for nursing as well as an effective trade union, that is what matters.

Time will tell.

EPILOGUE: THIS I BELIEVE

EPILOGUE: THIS I BELIEVE

Looking back over more than 50 years in nursing, I am proud of what I have been able to achieve, even though I have not always succeeded. I have always believed that if there are things you do not like about the world, you have to get out there and fight to change them. Sometimes you will not succeed and the wounds may be painful.

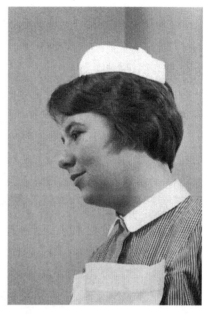

I can honestly say that I never fought alone. I owe a huge debt of gratitude to those whom, at the time, I did not even recognise as mentors, who were willing to nurture and invest in a 'wilful, pig-headed' young student, to support my outspokenness as a junior nurse, and to pick me up when I fell flat on my face. Without them I would not have had the amazing nursing journey I have had, nor would I have been as well positioned to give something back to a profession that has given so much to me. Nursing still is for me 'an exquisite obsession'.

As a member of the University Council, I recently attended Swansea University's graduation ceremony in the beautiful gold-ceilinged Brangwyn Hall. Garbed in my academic robes and with my Fellow of the RCN insignia on my chest, I sat on the platform, from where I could look down on the assembled new graduates and their guests. There were doctoral and masters awards in a range of health-related disciplines, but by far the most numerous were the graduating nurses. We celebrated, in the way Welsh people do, with speeches, poetry and song. For me, however, the highlight of the ceremony was when all the newly-graduating nurses were asked to stand to commit themselves to the pledge – an extract from the Nursing & Midwifery Council's Code of Practice.

Looking down on their fresh young faces, and listening to their enthusiasm as they responded to the Vice Chancellor's questions about what they were doing now and what they planned next, I swelled with pride.

There will always be people who need nursing, and I believe there will always be people who want to respond to that need.

As I watched, my mind wandered back to the day in October 1991 when a Service of Thanksgiving was held at Westminster Abbey to celebrate the RCN's diamond jubilee. Standing behind the great golden eagle lectern, I read the second lesson – not a biblical piece, but the 'Declaration of Belief about the Nature and Purpose of Nursing', taken from what is still my favourite book about nursing: Margretta Styles' *On Nursing: Toward a New Endowment*:

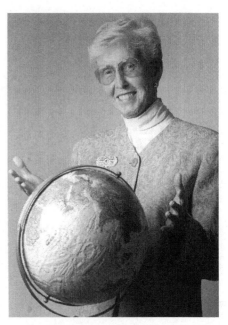

Margretta (Gretta) Styles

I believe in nursing as an occupational force for social good, a force that in the totality of its concern for all human health states and for mankind's responses to health and environment, provides a distinct, unique, and vital perspective, value orientation, and service.

I believe in nursing as a professional discipline requiring a sound education and research base grounded in its own science and in the variety of academic and professional disciplines with which it relates.

I believe in nursing as a clinical practice employing particular physiological, psychosocial, physical and technological means for human amelioration, sustenance, and comfort.

I believe in nursing as a humanistic field in which the fullness, self-respect, self-determination and humanity of the nurse engage the fullness, self-respect, self-determination and humanity of the client.

I believe that nursing's maximum contribution for social betterment is dependent upon:

- *The well-developed expertise of the nurse*
- *The understanding, appreciation and acknowledgement of that expertise by the public*
- *The organisational, legal, economic and political arrangements that engage the full and proper expression of nursing values and expertise*
- *The ability of the profession to maintain unity within diversity.*

I believe in myself and in my nursing colleagues:

- *in our responsibility to dedicate our minds, bodies, and souls to the profession that we esteem and the people whom we serve;*
- *in our right to be fulfilled, to be recognised, and to be rewarded as valued members of society.*

It was Gretta who first said 'Nursing is for me an exquisite obsession'. So it is for me.

The Clark family, August 2015

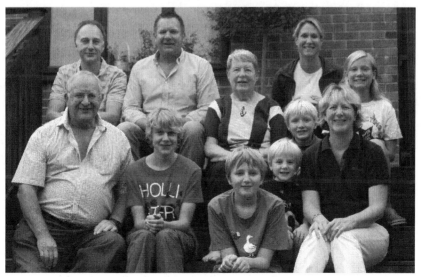

REFERENCES

American Nurses Association (1980) *Nursing: A Social Policy Statement.* American Nurses Association, Kansas City, MO

Antonovsky A (1979) *Health, Stress and Coping.* Jossey Bass Publishers, San Francisco, CA

Baly M, Robottom B, Clark J (1987) *District Nursing.* 2nd edn. Heinemann, London

Casey A, Clark J, Watterson L (2006) Are your indicators working? *Nurs Stand* **20**: 12–15

Clark J (1967) Whose fault? *Family Planning* **16**: 82–7

Clark J (1968) The new health visitor training 3: From a recent student's point of view. *Mother and Child* April: 11–14

Clark J (1969) It's different on the receiving end. *Nursing Mirror* 3 October: 30

Clark J (1969) Preparation for childbirth: A personal experience. *Nursing Times* **47**: 15–51

Clark J (1969) Learning for living. *Nursing Times* **47**: 181–2

Clark J (1970) Letters to the editor. *Nursing Times* **66**: 853–4

Clark J (1973) *A Family Visitor: A Descriptive Analysis of Health Visiting in Berkshire.* RCN, London

Clark J (1973) Diary of two babies: Ninth month. *Mother and Baby* February: 24

Clark J (1973) Diary of two babies; Tenth month. *Mother and Baby* March: 23

Clark J (1975) Diary of two babies; Thirty fourth month. *Mother and Baby* March: 35

Clark J (1976) The role of the health visitor: A study conducted in Berkshire, England. *J Adv Nurs* **1**: 25–36

Clark J (1976) Why I chose the RCN. *Nursing Mirror* **143**: 39–40

Clark J (1977) Functions and dysfunctions in a professional association: The case of the Royal College of Nursing. *J Adv Nurs* **2**: 299–310

Clark J (1978) *Family Health and Safety.* Queen Anne Press, London

Clark J (1979) The right to strike. *Nursing Mirror* **149**: 20–1

Clark J (1980) Where Clegg falls so short. *Nursing Mirror* 17 January: 8–10

Clark J (1980) *Premenstrual Tension.* Hamlyn Paperbacks, London

Clark J (1980) A framework for health visiting: Part 1: The application of systems theory to health visiting. *Health Visitor* **53**: 418–20

Clark J (1980) A framework for health visiting: Part 2: The nature of health visiting activity. *Health Visitor* **53**: 487–8

Clark J (1980) A framework for health visiting: Part 3: The environment and the time dimension. *Health Visitor* **53**: 533–5

Clark J (1982) Development of models and theories on the concept of nursing. *J Adv Nurs* **7**: 129–34

Clark J (1982) *What do Health Visitors do? A Review of the Research 1960–1980.* RCN, London

Clark J (1982) That uncertain knock at the door. *Nursing Mirror* **154**: 33–5

Clark J (1982) A way to get organised. *Nursing Times (Community Outlook)* 13 October (Suppl): 287–8 290, 295

Clark J (1984) Recording health visitor-client interaction in home visits. *Health Visitor* **57**: 5–8

Clark J (1985) Delivering the goods. *Nursing Times (Community Outlook)* January: 23–8

Clark J (1985) The process of health visiting. PhD thesis. CNAA. RCN Steinberg Collection, London

Clark J (1986) Free from the straitjacket. *Nursing Times* **66**: 28–9

Clark J (1991) Nursing: An intellectual activity. *BMJ* **303**: 376–7; reprinted in *Int Nurs Rev* (1991) **39**: 60

Clark J (1996) Information is power: How the ANA manages information. Unpublished report to General Secretary of the Royal College of Nursing

Clark J (1997) "The elements of nursing are all but unknown" Professorial Inaugural Lecture. University of Wales Swansea, Swansea

Clark J (1997) The unique function of the nurse. *Int Nurs Rev* **44**: 144–52 (Inaugural Virginia Henderson lecture)

Clark J (1998) The International Classification for Nursing Practice Project. *Online Journal of Issues in Nursing* 3: Manuscript 3. Available: www.nursingworld.org/MainMenuCategories/ANAMarketplace/ANAPeriodicals/OJIN/TableofContents/Vol31998/No2Sept1998/TheInternationalClassificationForNursingPracticeProject.aspx

Clark J (1998) The science of nursing. *Professional Nurse* **13**: 573

Clark J (1999) A language for nursing. *Nursing Standard* **13**: 42–7

Clark J (1999) An international perspective on nursing diagnosis development. In Rantz M, Le Mone P. *Classification of Nursing Diagnosis: Proceedings of the Thirteenth (NANDA) Conference.* Cinahl Information Systems, Glendale, CA

Clark J (2001) Meeting the challenge: the role of Fellows of the RCN. *Nursing Leadership Forum* **5**: 84–7

Clark J (ed) (2003) *Naming Nursing: Proceedings of the First ACENDIO Ireland/UK Conference held September 2003 in Swansea, Wales.* Verlag Hans Huber, Bern

Clark J (2006) 30th anniversary commentary on Henderson V (1978) The concept of nursing. *Journal of Advanced Nursing* 3, 113–130. *J Adv Nurs* **53**: 33–4

Clark J (2008) Ehealth: the human resources implications. In: *Commonwealth Health Ministers Book 2008.* Commonwealth Secretariat, London

Clark J, Buttigieg M, Bodycombe J et al (2000) *Recognising the Potential: A Review of Health Visiting and School Health Services in Wales.* University of Wales Swansea, Swansea

Clark J, Craft-Rosenberg M, Delaney C (2000) An international methodology to describe clinical nursing phenomena: a team approach. *Int J Nurs Stud* **37**: 541–53

Clark J, Christensen J, Mooney G et al (2001) New methods of documenting health visiting practice. *Community Practitioner* **74**: 108–11

Clark J, Henderson J (1983) *Community Health.* Churchill Livingstone, London

Clark J, Hiller RB (1975) *Community Care.* HMM Publishers, London

Clark J, Lang N (1992) Nursing's next advance: An international classification for nursing practice. *Int Nurs Rev* **39**: 109–12

Clay T (1987) *Nurses: Power and Politics.* Butterworth-Heinemann Ltd, London

Clinical Standards Advisory Group (1998) *Community Health Care for Elderly People.* The Stationery Office, London

Davidson A (1998) UK: The Davidson interview: Alan Langlands. *Management Today*, 1 February. Available: http://www.managementtoday.co.uk/news/411785/UK-Davidson-Interview---Alan-Langlands/?DCMP=ILC-SEARCH

Department of Health and Social Security and Scottish Home and Health Department (1972) *Report of the Committee on Nursing*. Cmnd 5115. HMSO, London (Briggs Report)

Department of Health and Social Security (1986) *Primary Health Care: An Agenda for Discussion*. Cmnd 9771. HMSO, London

Department of Health (1999) *Making a Difference: Strengthening the Nursing, Midwifery and Health Visiting Contribution to Health and Health Care*. DoH, London

Department of Health (2001) *Essence of Care*. DoH, London

Department of Health (1989) *Working for Patients: Education and Training (Working Paper 10)*. HMSO, London

Department of Health and Social Security (1968) *Report of the Committee on Local Authority and Allied Personal Social Services*. Cmnd 3703. HMSO, London (Seebohm Report)

Department of Health and Social Security (1972) *Management Arrangements for the Reorganised National Health Service*. HMSO, London

Department of Health and Social Security (1974) *Report of the Committee of Enquiry into the Pay and Related Conditions of Service of Nurses and Midwives*. HMSO, London (Halsbury Report)

Department of Health and Social Security (1981) *Growing Older*. HMSO, London

Department of Health and Social Security (1983) *NHS Management Enquiry*. DHSS, London (Griffiths Report)

Department of Health and Social Security (1986) *Neighbourhood Nursing: A Focus for Care*. HMSO, London (Cumberlege Report)

Goffman E (1961) *Asylums: Essays on the Social Situation of Mental Patients and Other Inmates*. Anchor Books, Garden City, NY

Henderson V (1960) *Basic Principles of Nursing Care*. International Council of Nurses, Geneva

Hughes R, Lloyd D, Clark J (2008) A conceptual model for nursing information. *Int J Nurs Terminol Classif* **19**: 48–56

Lowthian S (2015) Our strength is our members. *RCN Bulletin* **330**: 11

Mahler HA (1987) A powerhouse for change. *Senior Nurse* **6**: 23

McCormack B (1998) Community care for elderly people. *BMJ* **317**: 552–3

McGann S, Crowther A, Dougall R (2009) *A Voice for Nurses: A History of the Royal College of Nursing 1916–90*. Manchester University Press, Manchester

Menzies Lyth I (1960) Social systems as a defense against anxiety: An empirical study of the nursing servivice of a general hospital. *Human Relations* **13**: 95–121

Ministry of Health (1966) *Report of the Committee on Senior Nursing Staff Structure*. HMSO, London (Salmon Report)

National Assembly of Wales (1999) *Realising the Potential: A Strategic Framework for Nursing Midwifery and Health Visiting in Wales into the 21st Century*. National Assembly of Wales, Cardiff

National Assembly of Wales (2001) *Creating the Potential: A Plan for Education*. National Assembly of Wales, Cardiff

Parsonage S, Clark J (1981) *Infant Feeding and Family Nutrition*. HMM Publishers, London

Peate I (2013) Has the RCN lost its way? *Br J Nurs* **22**: 73

Rayner C (2003) *How Did I Get Here From There?* Virago, London

Rigby M, Roberts R, Williams J et al (1998) Integrated record keeping as an essential aspect of a primary care led health service. *BMJ* **317**: 579–82

Robb B (1967) *Sans Everything: A Case to Answer*. Nelson, London

Royal College of Nursing (1971) *Report of the Working Party on the Role of the Health Visitor Now and in a Changing National Health Service*. RCN, London

Royal College of Nursing (1974) *The State of Nursing*. RCN, London

Royal College of Nursing (1980) *Standards of Nursing Care*. RCN, London

Royal College of Nursing (1981) *Towards Standards*. RCN, London

Royal College of Nursing (1983) *Thinking About Health Visiting*. RCN, London

Royal College of Nursing (1984) *Accountability in Health Visiting*. RCN, London

Royal College of Nursing (1985) *The Education of Nurses: A New Dispensation*. RCN, London (Judge Report)

Royal College of Nursing (1987) RCN response to the consultation on primary health care initiated by the UK health departments. RCN, London

Royal College of Nursing (1990) *Quality Patient Care: The Dynamic Standard Setting System*. RCN, London

Royal College of Nursing (1992) *Powerhouse for Change: Report of the Taskforce on Community Nursing*. RCN, London

Royal College of Nursing (1992) *Powerhouse for Change: A Manifesto for Community Health Nursing in the 1990s*. RCN, London

Royal College of Nursing (2003) *Defining Nursing*. RCN, London

Royal College of Nursing (2006) *Putting Information at the Heart of Nursing Care: How IT is Set to Revolutionise Health Care and the NHS*. RCN, London

Royal Commission on Long Term Care, Sutherland S (1999) *With Respect to Old Age: Long Term Care – Rights and Responsibilities*. Cmnd 4192-I. The Stationery Office, London (Sutherland Report, Royal Commission on Long Term Care)

Royal Commission on the National Health Service (1979) *Royal Commission on the National Health Service* (Merrison Commission). Cmnd 7615. HMSO, London (Merrison Report)

Spinks M (2014) *From SRN to CBE: Celebrating 50 Remarkable Years in Nursing*. Quay Books, London

Standing Commission on Pay Comparability, Clegg H (1980) *Standing Commission on Pay Comparability Report No 3: Nurses and Midwives*. Cmnd 7795. HMSO, London

Styles MM (1982) *On Nursing: Toward a New Endowment*. CV Mosby, St Louis, MO

Tavistock Institute of Human Relations (1973) *An Exploratory Study of the RCN Membership Structure*. RCN, London

The Royal Society (2006) *Digital Healthcare: The Impact of Information and Communication Technologies on Health and Healthcare*. The Royal Society, London

UK Central Council for Nursing Midwifery and Heath Visiting (1986) *Project 2000: A New Preparation for Practice*. UKCC, London

Welsh Assembly Government (2003) *Fundamentals of Care: Guidance for Health and Social Care Staff*. Welsh Assembly Government, Cardiff

Welsh Assembly Government (2003) *Informing Healthcare*. Welsh Assembly Government, Cardiff

World Health Organization (1978) *Report of the International Conference on Primary Health Care, Alma Ata, USSR, 6–12 September 1978*. WHO, Geneva (Declaration of Alma-Ata)

World Health Organization (2000) *The Family Health Nurse: Context, Conceptual Framework, and Curriculum*. WHO, Copenhagen

World Health Organization (2001) *Second WHO ministerial Conference on Nursing and Midwifery in Europe Munich 15–17 June 2000*. WHO, Copenhagen

Other publications by June Clark (selected)

Books

Clark J (1973) *A Family Visitor: A Descriptive Analysis of Health Visiting in Berkshire*. RCN, London

Clark J, Hiller RB (1975) *Community Care*. HMM Publishers, London

Baly M, Robottom B, Clark J, Chapple M (1981) *A New Approach to District Nursing*. William Heineman Medical Books Ltd, London

Parsonage S, Clark J (1981) *Infant Feeding and Family Nutrition*. HMM Publishers, London

Clark J (1982) *What do Health Visitors do? A Review of the Research* 1960–1980. RCN, London

Clark J, Henderson J (1983) *Community Health*. Churchill Livingstone, London

Baly M, Robottom B, Clark J (1987) *District Nursing*. 2nd edn. Heinemann, London

Clark J, ed. (2003) *Naming Nursing: Proceedings of the First ACENDIO Ireland/UK Conference held September 2003 in Swansea, Wales*. Verlag Hans Huber, Bern

Chapters in edited books

Clark J (1974) The role of the health visitor. In: Bloomfield R, Follis P, eds. *The Health Team in Action*. BBC Publications, London

Clark J (1981) Theories on the concept of nursing. In: International Council of Nurses. *Health Care for All: Challenge for Nursing*. ICN, Geneva

Clark J (1986) A model for health visiting. In: Kershaw B, Salvage J, eds. *Models for Nursing*. John Wiley & Sons Ltd, London

Clark J (1992) An international classification for nursing practice: A challenge for nursing research. In: Krause K, Astedt-Kurki P, eds. *International Perspectives on Nursing*. University of Tampere Department of Nursing Publications, Tampere

Clark J (1993) Into the community. In: Dolan B, ed. *Project 2000: Reflection and Celebration*. Scutari Press, London

Clark J (1995) Nurses as managers. In: Baly M, ed. *Nursing and Social Change*. 3rd edn. Routledge, London

Clark J (1995) The road to reorganisation. In: Baly M, ed. *Nursing and Social Change*. 3rd edn. Routledge, London

Clark J (1995) Nursing research. In: Baly M, ed. *Nursing and Social Change*. 3rd edn. Routledge, London

Clark J (1996) Mapping our terrain: Developing a language and classification system for nursing practice. In: Lanara V, ed. *Quality in Nursing: Realities and Visions*. Nursing Society of Greece, Athens

Clark J (1997) Home care nursing in the United Kingdom. In: Modly D, Zanotti R, Poletti M, Fitzpatrick J, eds. *Home Care Nursing Services: International Lessons*. Springer, New York, NY

Clark J (1997) The International Classification for Nursing Practice. In: McCloskey JC, Grace HK, eds. *Current Issues in Nursing*. 5th edn. Mosby, St Louis, MO

Clark J (1999) An international perspective on nursing diagnosis. In: Rantz MJ, LeMone P, eds. *Classification of Nursing Diagnosis: Proceedings of the Thirteenth Conference. Celebrating the 25th Anniversary of NANDA*. Cinahl Information Systems, Glendale, CA

Clark J (2001) Health care and nursing education and practice in the United Kingdom. In: Dochertman JM, Grace HK, eds. *Current Issues in Nursing*. 6th edn. Mosby, St Louis, MO

Clark J (2004) New methods of documenting health visiting practice. In: Rigby M, ed. *Vision and Value in Health Information*. Radcliffe Medical Press Ltd, Oxford

Clark J (2006) Nursing in Britain: An overview of health care, nursing education and practice. In: Dochertman JM, Grace HK, eds. *Current Issues in Nursing*. 6th edn. Mosby, St Louis, MO

Clark J (2007) The essence of nursing. In: Hinchliffe S, Norman S, Schober J, eds. *Nursing Practice and Health Care*. Hodder Arnold, London

Clark J (2007) Nursing in an electronic world. In: Hinchliffe S, Norman S, Schober J, eds. *Nursing Practice and Health Care*. Hodder Arnold, London

Clark J (2007) The impact of ICT on health, healthcare and nursing in the next 20 years. In: Murray P, Park H-A, Erdley WS, Kim J, eds. *Nursing Informatics 2020: Towards Defining Our Own Future: Proceedings of the NI2006 Post Congress Conference, Volume 128 Stdies in Health Technology and Informatics*. IOS Press, Amsterdam

Clark J (2012) The United Kingdom's health system: Myths and realities. In: Mason DJ, Leavitt JK, Chaffee MW, eds. *Nursing Policy and Politics*. 6th edn. Elsevier, St Louis, MO